Radu's Simply Fit

Radu's Simply Fit

Enjoy the Workout of Your Life with America's Leading Fitness Coach

by Radu Teodorescu

with Maura Rhodes

Illustrations by Shawn Banner

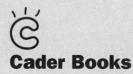

Cader Books

Andrews and McMeel
Kansas City

Thank you for buying this Cader Book—we hope you enjoy it. And thanks as well to the store that sold you this, and the hard-working sales rep who sold it to them. It takes a lot of people to make a book. Here are some of the many who were instrumental:

Editorial:
Camille N. Cline,
Jake Morrissey,
Dorothy O'Brien,
Regan Brown

Design:
Orit Mardkha-Tenzer

Cover design:
Charles Kreloff

Copy Editing/Proofing:
Miranda Ottewell,
Philip Reynolds,
Robert Legault

Production:
Carol Coe,
Cathy Kirkland

Legal:
Renee Schwartz, Esq.

**Cover and
Interior Photography:**
Frank Micelotta

If you would like to share any thoughts on this, or are interested in other books by us, write to:
**Cader Books
38 East 29th Street
New York, NY 10016**

Or visit our web site:
http://www.caderbooks.com

Library of Congress #96-83769
0-8362-1504-4 $18.95

July 1996

First edition

10 9 8 7 6 5 4 3 2 1

ATTENTION: SCHOOLS AND BUSINESSES
Andrews and McMeel books are available at quantity discounts with bulk purchase for educational, business, or sales promotional use. For information, please write to: Special Sales Department, Andrews and McMeel, 4520 Main Street, Kansas City, Missouri 64111.

I wish to express my love and gratitude to my wife, Victoria, and my two sons, Alexander and Andrew and thank them for helping me and coping with me.

I want to thank my mom, for understanding my preoccupation with this book during my last visit to Romania, which was my first after six years. All my love.

I also dedicate this book to all my professors and assistant professors at ICF, Bucharest (Physical Culture and Sports University), and especially to Professor and Rector of the University Mr. Dumitru Alexandrescu (née Mima) and Professor Barbu Victor.

And I wish give a heartfelt thanks to Nick Forstmann and Jackie Stewart for all their support.

Table of Contents

Surprise your muscles.

Acknowledgments

Special thanks go to Pamela Kawi, Karla Mayol, Eric Stiller, Gennadiy Shuminov, Alex-Aurel Astilean, Peter Janko, Jamie Miller, Eugene Rodda, Paul Deak, Debbie White, Roy Woelke, Christian Zarcu, Karen Hershkowitz, and Marian Grigoras for all their time, help, and support.

For supporting me in this endeavor, and, more importantly, inspiring me to be a better coach, I wish to give my very special thanks to Cindy Crawford, Regis Philbin, Al Roker, Matthew Broderick, Bianca Jagger, Matthew Modine, Vanessa Williams, and John Kennedy Jr.

And finally, thanks to all my students for sharing their feelings and ideas about Radu's method of training.

Radu's
Simply
Fit

A Simple Start

've been a trainer for over twenty years now, and in that time I've coached thousands of people from all walks of life, including dozens of celebrities. But ever since I started working with one particular model in 1988, all I've heard when new students come in or the press calls is, "Radu, I want my body to look like Cindy's."

Unfortunately only God and Mr. and Mrs. Crawford of Dekalb, Illinois, know how to pull that off. I didn't make Cindy Crawford what she is; I did help Cindy to make herself, though. That is what a good coach does. When she walked into my gym, Cindy was already beautiful, and she was already on her way to becoming one of the top models in the world. She had all of the raw talent, but like any champion she knew she needed a good coach to help push her to the top. Cindy was about to start work on a special project, a swimsuit calendar to benefit the National Leukemia Foundation (her brother had died of the disease at age three), and she wanted to show the world her absolute best. As any woman knows, looking good in a swimsuit is the ultimate physical challenge.

In the course of her training, Cindy went from looking beautiful to feeling beautiful, and to feeling great. After three months of hard and dedicated training, she lost some pounds and transformed herself into a leaner, more toned, and more accomplished physical machine. She became healthier, stronger, quicker, more flexible, and better coordinated every minute, with every move. And the calendar was a huge success. In the process, she also discovered athletic talents she never dreamed she had—for hiking, horseback riding, and even basketball. (She often challenges her good friend and mine, Regis Philbin, to a game of one-on-one when they're at my gym at the same time.) Cindy became a person who explores—a doer, an *athlete*.

Along the way she developed an immense self-confidence, a feeling of strength and rejuvenation, and the inner knowledge that her body isn't just something to be admired but something ready for action. She can project attitude while on skis, on ice skates, shooting hoops, and boxing, because she knows how. Learning to control and enjoy your body helps to get you centered, and that center holds solidly, no matter what life throws your way. As Cindy puts it, "The training transcended the physical. It taught me that I'm powerful—that I could conquer the world when I walk out of the gym."

This is what my approach does for people— rich and poor, famous and unknown alike. Now, with this book, I have a chance to welcome thousands more of you into my gym and into a world in which fitness and movement is exciting and your body becomes a source of pride and power— and you feel empowered for any challenge in your life. My program is about exercising your physical being, your will, and your spirit, all at the same time. It's about reaching back to the most basic and elemental physical building blocks, the pure and simple pleasures of asking your muscles to do something and getting

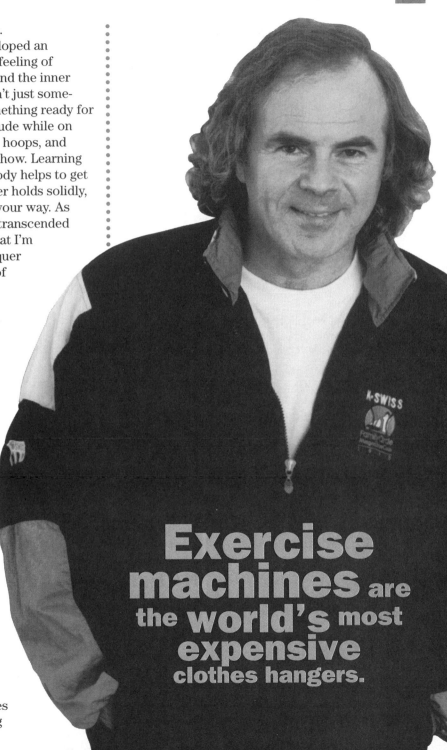

Exercise machines are the **world's** most **expensive** clothes hangers.

Never forget there's an even better you just over the horizon.

fluid, easy, and instant results. But it's also about reaching back to the vibrancy and innocence of childhood, when you enjoyed running and jumping and throwing without thinking about it or making it into work. It's about giving you the feeling, and the tools, to do anything, anywhere. It's about preparing your body and mind to work together, and it's about preparing for life.

If you think this sounds ambitious, you're right, but if you think that this means that my program is complicated, then you're wrong. If you think about it for a minute, you'll realize that a lot of what people today call "exercise" doesn't make much good common sense. There's no reason that we should need fancy machines and exotic theme-routines to get our bodies in shape. If that's what human beings required for existence, we never would have made it this far up the evolutionary chain. The exercises I like best are the ones that are instinctively familiar to your muscles, that your body recognizes and responds to, that evoke the movement and work you do every day, and that your body remembers from its most enjoyable moments.

The simple truth is that when Cindy works out with me, she climbs, throws,

catches, skips, hops, and runs. And she shoots hoops outside my office door, climbs the ropes that hang from my ceiling, and swings and stretches on my high bar. She works hard, and she sweats hard, and occasionally she even complains a little bit. And sure, depending upon what she wants to focus on, I throw in some isolated movements, many of which you will find later in this book in a special section that highlights some of her special workout routines. But what I do with Cindy, and with all my students, is to put together basic, fun routines and exercises that challenge the body in the purest and simplest way and help all of the muscles to work in concert. I fill my students with a positive focus, a set of goals to shoot for, so that they understand that exercise is not an end in and of itself but a means to a more active, more enjoyable life. This is getting fit simply.

And this is what happens every day in my gym on West 57th Street in New York City and this is what can happen for you with this book in hand. Let me tell you, my studio is no health club—it's a gym. When people come to me they come to work out. This is not a social club or a place to check out the latest trends in spandex. We do the work, and we share the fun and exhilaration that comes with doing work well.

A lot of people say my studio reminds them of their high-school gym, and with good reason. We have a polished wooden floor with basketball hoops, flanked by walls with ropes and ladders for climbing. There are medicine balls and free weights and some minimal weight-training equipment—and yes, a couple of exercise machines for specific needs. But if we're doing stairs as part of the day's workout, we head up the stairwell in my building, just the way you probably did in high school (can you imagine a principal spending money on machines that simulate stairs?). My program is fundamentally nothing more than phys ed class for grown-ups. In fact, the name of my studio is Radu's Physical Culture, which helps to communicate my mission of educating people about their bodies. Back when you were in school you couldn't imagine that movement and sports and sweating would ever cease to be a natural part of your life. So you never paid much attention to the educational aspect of phys ed, you just went and shook the day's demons out of your body and went back to class a little bit tired and little bit rejuvenated. On the most fundamental level, I'm not a trainer, I'm a teacher, and the goal of my classes is to help people learn to live better.

The Big Secret

I recently celebrated my fiftieth birthday at a wonderful party thrown for me by friends Cindy and Regis. I've been in the fitness business for 27 years, which is saying something pretty amazing, since most people think of this as a young person's field. For all those years, legions of fitness journalists, other trainers, and celebrities have flocked to my gym, and they still come. As I have just told you, they're not coming for the fancy facilities or the luxurious extras; they come because of the simple and compelling effectiveness of my approach.

I know that there are plenty of fitness books and videos out there, plenty of them by so-called "trainers to the stars," offering body-shaping "secrets." Don't get me wrong, I'm glad that you may have picked up my book because you know what I've done for Cindy or Regis or Matthew Broderick and you're hoping that maybe I can do the same for you. So let me tell you the biggest training secret of all right now and get the suspense out of the way: There are no training secrets.

The fundamentals of fitness are really pretty simple. It's all about good honest work. Muscle is primary. You work the muscles, and you try to work them evenly and thoroughly, and they get stronger. The best exercises of all are the simplest, most straightforward ones that work the muscle groups you mean to be working. Anything beyond that is really just a gimmick. And the odds are that any gimmick that excites people today will be forgotten tomorrow.

The real secret to my training is attitude. Training is just that—preparation. Preparation for everything else in your life, whether it's walking up the four flights of stairs to your apartment, carrying around your toddler, bicycling around the park, or climbing a cliff to enjoy the spectacular view that you can only get by scaling it yourself. We all know that exercise is good for us, and yet the overwhelming majority of Americans don't do it. The whole key is motivating yourself to get up and go exercise.

Exercise in and of itself will always be boring and tedious. If all you can do is some repetitive movements in a stuffy room, if you never get a chance to enjoy what you can do with your body, then exercise will always be a burden to you. As exercise becomes a burden—something you make yourself do instead of something you want to do—then fitness is left by the wayside, instead of an essential part of a healthy and well-rounded life. But exercise that is a part of your life, a component of preparing for everything else in your life, is the groundwork that lets you do everything you want to do.

The point of training is to prepare yourself for all of the fun things that you can do once you are trained. And that is how exercise can and will transform your life in a dramatic fashion. Not because you can spin around at level 8 on an imitation bicycle or climb a hundred flights on an electronic staircase—no real sense of fun or accomplishment goes with that. But when you can play an hour of full-court basketball without getting winded, or climb a mountain that you could never get on top of, or see the countryside from the seat of a bicycle, or kayak waters that you were afraid to set foot in, then you are reaping the true benefits, and only then has exercise done something to improve your life.

When John Kennedy Jr. comes to train with me, it's not because he's looking for a new girlfriend or trying to fit into a new suit. It's because he loves going on adventures. He's always looking to raise his fitness level to help him meet a new challenge. One time it was for a biking trek; another for a kayaking trip in the Red Sea. He'll tell me what new journey he's getting ready for, and I'll put together a quick program to help get him ready (see his arm and shoulder exercises in Personal Training on pages 77–79). He is so motivated by his ultimate goal that then he can go off and train himself with no problem.

I always emphasize to my students these positive benefits of thorough training. Too many fitness programs focus on losing a certain number of pounds, or changing how one part of the body looks, or worst of all, struggling to live a little longer. Now there's a happy goal that really gets you motivated to put on your exercise clothes. While for many people these goals are valid, they're ultimately unsatisfying as final aims for a training program. You drop a few pounds, and then what? You are out of goals, you lose interest in your program, and pretty soon you are back where you

started. This is the yo-yo that plagues dieters and exercisers alike. The student whose limited goals and attitude I can't change is the student who will never stay with her program or make a lasting change in her life.

I've been told that my brand of training is visible on just about anyone I work with. A good friend of mine once commented about a benefit she attended where a number of my students were also present. My friend said, "You know, there were a lot of great-looking people at the party, but it was so easy to tell who had been trained by Radu. They held themselves differently, they stood taller, they *glowed* with energy."

Much of that radiance and confidence comes from the fact that my training method is multidimensional. My program focuses on the standard four fundamental physical qualities—strength, speed, endurance, and flexibility—plus my own special fifth quality, balance and coordination, which adds agility. Leave out just one of these elements, and you have a body that is pretty fit, almost fit, but by no means *completely* fit. The actors, models, and well-known and not-yet-known personalities who come to my gym do so because they get the confidence that they will look great no matter who is looking or where the camera is positioned. When a model trains with me I give her the streamlined body she needs for the camera—but I also give her the confidence she needs for the runways. An actor gets the physical capabilities to play a part and perform a stunt, but he also gets the attitude to carry it off and make the stunt a believable accomplishment for his character.

I don't believe exercise should be a mindless activity. The body and mind can't work well separately from each other. To the contrary, I try to make exercise a mindful activity. I don't let Cindy or any of my students just come in and do what I say for an hour without giving them reasons why. And I want you to be able to take what you learn in these pages about movement and activity and use that knowledge whenever and wherever you find yourself.

All You Need To Know About Fitness You Learned In Phys Ed

Ever since Robert Fulghum wrote his famous book about the simple truths learned in childhood, many people have been working on making their lives less complicated and looking for the simple truths. Now the search for simplicity is a trend all by itself. As far as I am concerned, that's great. After all, don't you find it mind-boggling that we need to do so much *stuff* to stay in shape? No wonder people talk about going to "work out." Exercise should feel like play; who needs to go looking for more work?

So let's call it playing; now don't you want to join in? Of course, to play you have to know the rules and develop the right skills. When you were a kid, you never realized that your play was also exercise—it was fun and spontaneous and totally natural. You were not embarrassed to chase a ball or miss a shot. Kids are lean and agile because they know how to have fun with their bodies without anyone telling them—they run and jump and climb, and they are flexible without having to work at it. You didn't think about it, and you never thought of it as exercise. Have you ever seen a toddler run down the sidewalk? Try imitating that same whole-body run and you'll

exhaust yourself within minutes. When I go climbing with my two children, they sprint to the top before my wife and I can barely get started.

The sad truth is that an average adult's life isn't as active and physically demanding as it used to be. With laziness and complacency, we've only made it worse on ourselves. I know many people whose idea of an adventuresome weekend in the "country" is driving to the Hamptons, breathing the "fresh air" from an open convertible, going to cocktail parties, networking with colleagues, looking at the beach through the window, and driving back to the city in bumper-to-bumper traffic. That's their great weekend outdoors.

It used to be that we didn't have to think about taking care of our bodies, because we used them every day just to survive. Can you imagine a group of cavemen organizing an aerobics class? Up until very recently, life itself was a physical struggle. Even in the early stages of industrialization, people still walked to work, climbed stairs, did heavy labor, and more. Now computers and machines have taken over much of the physical work, and the so-called "service economy" has taken a lot of the ordinary everyday labor of carrying and fixing and maintaining out of our lives as well. So we

There needs to be "ed" in phys ed.

spend a lot of time inventing new machines and new exercises that offer high-tech simulations of what our ancestors did naturally every day. Not only is the spontaneity gone, but we expect new developments and new machines to keep making exercise interesting for us.

In a vicious cycle, machines create a dependency that will prevent you from exercising whenever you can't get to wherever the equipment is, or when it breaks down. (I know a lot of writers who have become so dependent upon computers that they can't write when their computers are broken.) And no matter how many bells and whistles a machine has, it can never imitate the complexity of natural human movement (*"just like* walking," the ads say, or, *"just like* cross-country skiing"). You can't train exclusively on a treadmill and then one day decide to go outside to run: your heart and lungs will be fine, for a while, but your legs will give out because they are used to moving only on a flat surface at a specific speed. Your legs haven't been challenged by the random and natural changes in terrain, incline, wind speed, and temperature of the outdoors.

The only failure is the person who doesn't try.

By contrast, my program requires little equipment, and it gives so much by way of simplicity and fun that it is easy to stick with year after year. Once you've started you'll be amazed that you ever stopped. Activity is a necessity of life; you crave it as much as sleeping and eating. Once you recognize that craving, then you can start to feed it.

What Are They Really Like?

When I first opened my studio, it was a small, exclusive place that for almost five years was pretty much the secret province of celebrities. And ever since, actors, models, singers, and athletes have made up a big part of my clientele. My first well-known students were people like the designer Halston and the movie director Joel Schumacher, as well as others like Willi Smith, Tony Bennett, Susan Sarandon, Bianca Jagger, and Ben Gazzara, to name a few. These people were leading fast-paced lives, working hard by day and partying hard around the clock.

This was the disco era, when fitness meant increasing the ability to perform—at work and on the dance floor. Going to a gym to work out with a coach was a pretty new idea back then. Jogging was the big national exercise. (Some people even treated jogging like a drug, working themselves to exhaustion to get the "high" of their endorphins kicking in.) It wasn't until the late 1970s and early 1980s that disco-mania flowered into the whole aerobics movement and large numbers of people became more interested in their overall fitness. The unfortunate truth is that, as a friend of mine suggested, in those days the motto of my gym should have been, "If you want to do drugs, train with Radu." There would have been lines of people outside my door had I adopted that slogan.

So you can see what I was up against. Perhaps celebrities were attracted to me at first because they were some of the highest livers of all. They, more than anyone else at the time, were seeking an almost unreasonable level of performance around the clock, and even when some turned to drugs for recreation, they knew that real power and real endurance would have to come from their bodies, not from artificial stimulation.

As I noted before, my real mission is to spread the joy and pleasure of exercise to as many people as possible. But celebrities seem to like what I do for them, and they remain a big part of my clientele. The biggest challenge I face now with the stars sent by movie studios and production companies is that they always come in and say, "I just have to look great in three weeks." When someone like Anthony Quinn comes to me and says "Hey, Radu, I'm going to play Zorba the Greek on Broadway and I have to drop some pounds," I get a little crazy; you don't have to be a director to know that a good performance requires more than just a slimmer torso. I knew he was going to be performing a physically challenging role on stage night after night. Tony resisted me every step of the way at the beginning. He is as hotheaded as I am. I'd yell, he'd yell louder. I'd say, "Do this, do that!" He'd say, "Who the hell do you think you are?" And I'd get him every time: "I'm your *coach!*" Because in Radu's gym, Radu is the boss; nobody gets off easy, no matter who they are, but everyone thanks me for it later. And Tony gave great performances, exuding power, stamina, and agility.

You won't get off easy either. You will definitely thank me for it later. Of course, you won't have me around to shout at you if you start dropping the ball, so I need your attention now so that you can concentrate on both the message and the content of this book. Because without the message, my program is little more than just another sequence of exercises. I want you to hear my voice when you work out; I want you to sense my encouragement and support. And I want to you visualize what you are doing for yourself, where you are going, and how much better you are going to feel and how much more you are going to be able to do. I need you to see yourself climbing that mountain on your bike, or soaring to the basket when your opponent is out of steam, or catching that drop shot at the net that you could never reach before. And if it helps, you can see yourself like many of the celebrities who came to see me and survived, and who still think of me and hear my voice when they are conquering a physical challenge of their own. You will join the ranks of celebrities who continue to thank me, like Raquel Welch, Tuesday Weld, Debbie Gibson, Rita Moreno, Tatum O'Neal, Faye Dunaway, John Cusack, Calvin Klein, and Natasha Richardson. Jennifer Grey followed in the footsteps of her dad Joel, doing gymnastics in my gym before she became famous in *Dirty Dancing*. Supermodels like Cindy and Vendela and many others have shared my court with world-class athletes like Vitas Gerulaitis, Mark Breland, Michael McCallum, Evander Holyfield, and Riddick Bowe.

Regis Philbin and I started with a student-coach relationship that has grown into a lasting friendship. We first met when I was hired to help Regis develop "washboard abs"—a New Year's resolution that started as a fun gimmick on his morning talk show,

Live with Regis and Kathie Lee. But as he started working with me, Regis developed a real love for fitness, and now he and I go through an impressive full regimen together. But Regis is tough on me too (including giving me grief about not getting my hair cut for the cover of this book). He demands excellence—which I like. Sometimes guests on the show are students of mine, like Bronson Pinchot, and they'll start swapping war stories about me with Regis. Some people even say that my thick Romanian accent was part of the inspiration for the voice of Bronson's character Balki on *Perfect Strangers*; he liked to imitate me a lot when he was working on the role.

My students do develop a kinship—the same way soldiers in boot camp do. They come together by talking about how tough it was and how glad they are they survived the drill sergeant—but deep down they know they are better, stronger, more disciplined, and more capable than they ever believed they could be when they first appeared on my doorstep.

So what are all these celebrities really like? When it comes to fitness, they are just like you. They're a little scared, a little out of shape, and at least a little bit motivated to do something about it. They usually start with a limited goal, and with my help they begin to realize how big they can dream, and how much they can accomplish, and how good it feels to have a body that works the way a body should.

Tough Love

A lot of people, from my friend Regis to the editors of *New York* magazine, often talk about how tough I am (*New York* actually dubbed me the Toughest Trainer in Town, and the nickname stuck.) Often, though, people find my program "tough" because it challenges, and trains, the entire body as a unit. Plenty of people, including other trainers, come to my gym thinking they are in good shape. What they discover is that selected parts of their bodies may be in good shape, but they aren't well developed all over. Ultimately, you are only as strong as your weakest part. That's why I believe in total conditioning. I don't want to fool you; getting fit, even with the right attitude, the right trainer, and the right program, still involves a lot of serious work. The rewards are great, but you've got to do the work to collect the pay.

Added to that, personal experience has taught me that coddling is not the way to get results. In Romania, I played all sorts of sports. As a teenager I was on soccer, handball, and track-and-field teams, and I excelled at gymnastics. I graduated from the Physical Culture University of Bucharest, one of the most highly regarded schools for sports training and physical education in the world. Bela Karolyi, the famous gymnastics coach, graduated from there, as did his protégée Nadia Comaneci, plus athletes and coaches like Ilie Nastase and Ion Tiriac. I taught phys ed at a high school for three years, but things in Communist Romania at the time were very bad, and after seeing Jane Fonda's *They Shoot Horses, Don't They?* in 1972, I decided to escape the country.

I entered a political asylum program in Italy, but was arrested by police at the Austrian border when I tried to leave. They sent me to Vienna. Finally I went to the American embassy there and was granted permission to enter the United States. I arrived in America with little more than the clothes on my back. I washed dishes by day and worked as a security guard at night. I attended courses at the University of Bridgeport in Connecticut and at Hunter College in New York City so that I could teach physical education in this country. Eventually, I became a trainer, first at Nicholas Kounovsky's gym in Manhattan, and later at the Alex and Walter Exercise Studio, which catered to many famous people.

My real dream has always been to motivate masses of people to become healthier and happier through exercise; I want everyone to experience the joy of movement. I slowly realized that none of the very specific training methods my employers had me executing were good enough, or well rounded enough, to give my students the performance and the fitness they were after, or to provide the kind of physical satisfaction I was after. This turned out to be a very liberating revelation; my bosses didn't understand what I was talking about, and that motivated me to prove my methods to the world. I opened my own gym on October 19, 1977; it was my birthday, and exactly five years from when I set sail for America. My celebrity students were quickly drawn to my contagious enthusiasm and the exclusivity of my gym, but the rich and famous kept Radu's Physical Culture a secret until around 1983. I had been in business for five years.

Now I have two gyms, one in Manhattan and another in East Hampton, Long Island. In addition, I have created fitness programs at health clubs and at spas such as Safety Harbor Spa and Fitness Center in Tampa, Florida, and the Greenhouse in Arlington, Texas. I have served as an honorary national chairman for Workout for Hope since 1993, a fund-raising program sponsored each year by City of Hope, a nonprofit organization dedicated to AIDS and related cancer research.

Still, I feel my crusade is just getting started. But I know that this is my gift, and my purpose in life. And I've come to realize the profound effect that my training has had on people. A wall on my gym is filled with countless letters, snapshots, and postcards from all kinds of students—testaments to the amazing obstacles they have gone on to conquer, their achievements, and a sense of bliss that they attribute to their work with me. The celebrity testimonials you can read at the back of this book are just a tiny representation of what I hear from people all of the time. Some of my students have been with me since 1977 and are still going strong. Nothing gives me greater satisfaction than seeing people truly turn their lives around by discovering the power within themselves, the ability to greet the world around them with a zest for adventure, and the confidence to prosper.

No matter the reasons, I'm glad that you have found your way to my gym. I will restore the simplicity and fun of fitness to you in the pages of this book. Exercise involves learning, practicing, and mastering certain skills, but it is also enjoyable. Working out will become more satisfying for you, as it is for me, and you will know that while you're having such a terrific time, you're also getting what some people only achieve through dreaded hard work and expensive health club dues. You'll be getting fit, simply.

The Plan

Just like any other sport, fitness is a game, and it requires a solid game plan. You need to set goals and establish a sequence of moves and plays to get you to those goals. And of course you already have me as a strong coach to guide you every step of the way.

After all, how you can expect to have a transformative experience when you don't have a plan for getting there, or even know what "there" is? You need to know where you're starting from and what you want to achieve. You also want to make certain that your first encounters with exercise are positive ones: you shouldn't ask so much of yourself at the beginning that you feel discouraged from the start. My goal is clear: to give you all the tools, the knowledge, and the motivation it takes to make exercise a permanent priority, a life-sustaining habit.

If you are new to exercise, you may want to spend a few days or even a week just getting used to working out in small doses before you attempt the entire basic Class that follows this chapter. Start your program each morning after you wake up. Stretch like a cat, touch your toes, run in place. Do a few jumping jacks, push-ups, sit-ups, squats—without worrying about how many. In fact, don't do this for more than ten to fifteen minutes. Mostly, you are getting yourself started on a habit; once you get used to it, you'll start to miss it if you don't keep to your program.

Whether or not you are new to fitness, you need to complete the following simple written exercise: Draw a line down the middle of a long piece of paper. Label the column on the left "Goals," the column on the right "Obstacles." Write down everything you would like to achieve in the next few years. I do mean everything—not just physical goals, but those pertaining to your career, your love life, your desire to master the piano or learn a second language or write a novel. The goals can be as large—to fly a plane—or as small—to break your nail-biting habit—as you wish. For the larger goals, break them down into the stages you need to achieve in order to reach the final goal. In the Obstacles column, write down what you perceive to be the thing preventing you from achieving each goal. Spend a lot of time on this; take a few days if you need to.

Once you're satisfied with your list, look over the obstacles. Which are genuine? If all that is preventing you from reaching a certain goal are minor obstacles, perhaps that goal isn't high enough. Among the major obstacles, do you notice a common denominator? Are these obstacles that have been placed in your path, or are they really self-imposed? Could it be that you're standing in your own way?

I want you to look at all of the goals in your life, because the same drive to achieve that applies in the gym applies in the real world. If you learn how to achieve one goal—regardless of whether it pertains to exercise, work, or your personal life—then accomplishing others will follow naturally. And one goal leads to another; in fitness this is especially true if you take it a step at a time. Cindy Crawford achieved so much through exercise, she felt empowered to move on and reach other goals in her life. When you see—and feel—that you have achieved something, when you experience the joy of that achievement, you will only want more.

The Simplest Fitness Test You'll Ever Take

Physical progress can be measured in many ways. The best ruler is the most natural one:

your energy level, your zest for life, your need and pleasure in making exercise a priority every single day, your interest in participating in sports, and your appreciation for opportunities to interact with nature and your teammates. These qualities are the most meaningful measure because they indicate the way toward some of the most meaningful rewards of getting fit.

Nonetheless, it is nice to have some awareness of the more objective aspects of your achievements as well—pounds and inches lost or gained if your aim is to shape certain body parts, increases in the number of repetitions you can do, and so on. Noting your activity daily and taking the evaluation every month on the charts provided (photocopy these as necessary for future use) will give you a tangible picture of your fitness and health gains, and it will help you to figure out when you're ready to make changes in your program. If you find that after doing the basic Class for several months you hit a plateau—you don't experience measurable changes—then you should consider adding new exercises to your program from the Personal Training routines (most of which pinpoint specific muscle groups), or moving on to the Ultimate Challenge. Likewise, you will only see the tangible results if you complete the basic Class three to four times per week. It is important to have the proper clothing, equipment, and instruction before you begin exercises or activities of any kind.

Finally, before you start, make sure you're in good health. These are not rehabilitation routines for the injured or disabled: they're designed for people who have no chronic health problems, such as asthma, heart disease, diabetes, epilepsy, or hemophilia, or physical anomalies, like knee pain or back or neck trouble, that might be exacerbated by activity. If in doubt, have a thorough checkup first.

Getting Started

Before you start your exercise program, fill out the chart below by taking your measurements as indicated in parentheses and completing the individual tests that follow on pages 16–17. This evaluation will help you determine your baseline. Be sure to record your results once a month thereafter to get a sense of your progress.

BODY MEASUREMENTS	Baseline	Month 1	Month 2	Month 3	Month 4
WEIGHT					
CHEST (measure across nipple and the shoulder blade)					
WAIST (measure at narrowest point)					
HIPS (measure with feet together, at widest point)					
THIGHS: Left/Right (measure at widest point, just below buttocks)	/	/	/	/	/
UPPER ARMS: Left/Right (measure with arm extended, palm up)	/	/	/	/	/

FITNESS TESTS (see p. 16–17 for instructions)	Baseline	Month 1	Month 2	Month 3	Month 4
PUSH-UPS					
SIT-UPS					
SQUATS					
ENDURANCE					
UPPER BODY FLEXIBILITY					
LOWER BODY FLEXIBILITY					
BALANCE AND COORDINATION					

	Month 5	Month 6	Month 7	Month 8	Month 9	Month 10	Month 11	Month 12
	/	/	/	/	/	/	/	/
	/	/	/	/	/	/	/	/

	Month 5	Month 6	Month 7	Month 8	Month 9	Month 10	Month 11	Month 12

Fitness Tests

Complete these seven tests and record the results on the previous chart.

PUSH-UPS

This is a measure of your upper-body strength. You may do a standard push-up (legs straight) or a modified push-up (on hands and knees, ankles crossed and off the floor.) Do as many repetitions as you can, making sure that your chest comes within three inches of the floor.

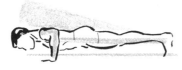

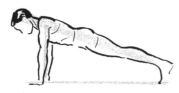

Standard: Place your hands on the floor about shoulder-width apart, fingers pointing forward. Extend your legs behind you, feet together and balanced on toes. Make sure your head is in line with your spine. Tighten your abs and tuck your pelvis so that your body is straight. Keeping your body stiff as a board, bend your elbows until your chest is just a few inches from the floor, then return to starting position.

Modified: Kneel on hands and knees, hands shoulder-width apart, fingers facing forward. Bring your feet off the floor, tuck your pelvis, and tighten your knees. Bend your elbows until your chest is just a few inches from the floor, then return to starting position.

SIT-UPS

This evaluates the strength of your abdominals. You may need a partner to hold your ankles, or you can anchor your feet under a chair or lie on your back, knees bent, feet apart. Bend your elbows close to your sides, hands fisted. Sit up, straightening your arms past your legs. Your shoulders should touch down each time your return to starting position. Count the number of sit-ups you can do within one minute.

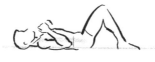

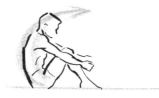

SQUATS

To test the strength of your lower body, you can do either full squats or half-squats. Stand in front of a sturdy chair with your hands on your thighs; squat until you're almost sitting on the chair, then return to starting position. Count the number you can complete until exhaustion or within a minute.

ENDURANCE

This is a measure of the health of your cardiovascular system—your aerobic health. You will need a sturdy, eight- to twelve-inch-high platform, step or bench, and a timer (preferably a wristwatch that beeps so you don't have to keep an eye on it). Set the timer for three minutes and begin stepping up and down off the bench at the rate of twenty-four steps a minute. Stop as soon as the three minutes have passed, sit down and keep your eye on the clock. Begin counting your pulse exactly thirty seconds after sitting; count for thirty seconds. This number is your recovery heart rate.

FLEXIBILITY

Upper Body: Sit up straight. Raise your left arm and then bend your elbow so that your hand lands between your shoulder blades. At the same time, reach behind your back with your right arm, bending the elbow and attempting to bring your right fingers in contact with your left. If your fingertips do not touch, have someone measure the distance between them, then try the test in the opposite direction, again measuring the results.

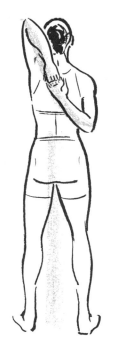

Lower Body: Grab a yardstick and sit down on an uncarpeted floor. Extend your legs in front of you, with your feet approximately twelve inches apart. Lay the ruler on the floor between your legs, with the thirty-six-inch mark away from you, the one-inch mark between your legs, and your heels aligned with the fifteen-inch mark. Flex your feet and extend your arms straight in front of you, hands flat and one on top of the other, palms down, and fingers aligned. Exhale and reach forward as far as you can, allowing your head to relax forward and your fingers to touch the stick. Note where your fingers touch (in inches). Repeat the test three times; the farthest point you reach indicates your flexibility.

BALANCE AND COORDINATION

Stand on your right leg, extend both arms out to the side, and lift your left leg into the air behind you. Time how long you can maintain this position, then repeat with the other leg.

Simply Fit
Terminology

Load
The amount of weight (kg. or lb.) used.

Reps (repetitions)
The basic motion of an exercise.

Set
A group of reps.

Rotation
A group of sets.

Intensity
Refers to quality—the maximum amount of resistance overcome through muscular contraction.

Volume
Refers to quantity—amount of work performed during a session.

Rest Period
Refers to your recovery rate—the time it takes for heart rate to come down to the working plateau (plateau reached after a full warm-up but before exercise section). Complete recovery occurs after the cool-down section.

Cardio (cardiovascular) Training
Emphasizes endurance through heart, lung, and muscle conditioning.

Athletic Training
Emphasizes performance in different sports. Also relates to various systems of training, including interval and fartlek (see below).

General Conditioning
Preparation for all kinds of activities, including sports and recreation.

Physical Education
Learning the basic human movements needed in life.

Cosmetic
Refers to body building—the only system that does not address performance or efficiency because it is based upon isolated movements.

Interval Training
An athletic method of training that alternates sprints of 30, 50, 110, and 440 yards with rest periods of 60 to 90 seconds.

Fartlek Training
An athletic method of training that alternates intensity from fast to slow and intersperses this pattern with altering direction.

The Daily Log

The best way to gauge your overall progress is by monitoring your daily exercise. By charting your physical ups and downs, and reviewing them at the end of each day, week, or couple of weeks, you'll be able to understand more fully the results of your monthly tests and body measurements. The activities you include in your Daily Log should not only center on the classes and additional exercises in this book, but should also include any outdoor sports and extra exercise—helping friends move or refereeing youth basketball—you get throughout the course of your day.

The Daily Log is your exercise journal. Your entries will range from recording the number of Class push-up sets you were really able to finish to what you ate for lunch to the amount of time you spent riding your bike the same day. The following descriptions will help you create your daily training log.

TYPE OF PROGRAM: As you progress through the Class in the next chapter, you will begin to add specific exercises for specific body parts from Personal Training. And after you've mastered your customized Class, you will move on to the Ultimate Challenge and eventually add specific exercises to it also; for example, "The Ultimate Challenge, plus Vanessa Williams' Personal Training exercises."

REPS/SETS/LOAD: Every day you will exercise differently, even if you are doing the same program. In fact, I encourage you to vary your routine as you become comfortable with it. Write down the reps, sets, or amount of weight you were able to do.

ADDITIONAL ACTIVITY: Apply your newfound fitness to the world outside your training space. Exercises from the Class, Personal Training, and the Ultimate Challenge prepare you for the activities you really want to improve at, like biking longer, swimming farther, playing volleyball with greater skill, or anything you've dreamed of doing but could not do before. Log that day's sport or activity, the distance you crossed (in miles, laps, flights of stairs), and the time you spent.

YOUR DAILY EVALUATION: After describing your programs and additional activities, describe how you feel. Say you just did three sets of ten reps each of forward lunges. Was the last rep harder than the first two? Easier? Did you feel the stretch? Did you keep your balance on every rep? Or say you just completed the marathon you'd been training for. How was the start? Did you hit a wall at the end? How did you overcome it?

Here is an example of a Daily Log:

THURSDAY:

6:30 Slept well. Skipped breakfast.

7:00–8:00 Did the Class, plus Regis Philbin's head crushers: did all sets, intermediate reps, except when I got to weights. Did one set of beginning reps for weights and used lightest weight for each exercise. Added head crushers after pullovers in rotation. Diamond and pretzel stretch felt great.

1:00–2:00 Light lunch and did the running sequence from Time-Efficient Program in my office.

6:00–7:30 Played softball with corporate league after work; sprinted the bases almost every other inning.

8:30–10:00 Lugged groceries up two flights, had a full dinner, and finished painting bathroom.

Weight Training Basics

When you're working with weights, as many of my exercises call for, there are certain basic rules you should follow to make sure you get the most out of the moves and to prevent injury. You'll need several sets of dumbbells (good starting weights are three, five, and eight pounds for a woman; five, eight, ten, and twelve for a man).

MAINTAIN PROPER FORM. Follow the description and illustration of the exercise you're doing. Even the body parts that you aren't moving are being used to balance and stabilize you, so you need to always keep your form.

MOVE THROUGH A FULL RANGE OF MOTION. In other words, open the joint you're using as far as it will go, and do not stop short when returning to starting position. Otherwise, you'll work the muscle to only a fraction of its capacity. You can also increase the effectiveness of any move by resisting the pull of gravity as you return to starting position. Lower the weight slowly and in a controlled manner.

SUSTAIN A FLUID PACE in proportion to the range of motion, degree of difficulty, and amount of weight. Move slowly and deliberately when hefting heavy weights. Don't go so fast that momentum, rather than muscle strength, is moving the weight.

BREATHE PROPERLY. Exhale as you lift the weight and inhale as you return to starting position. When alternating weights, time your breathing to just one arm's lift so that you're exhaling and inhaling rhythmically.

MATCH WEIGHT TO FITNESS LEVEL. For each exercise, there is a correct weight to use for your level of fitness. To figure this out, try each exercise using various weights. Use the weight at which you can complete a full set of ten repetitions; the last three should require concentration and effort. Write your starting weight down in your first Daily Log.

WHEN YOU BEGIN EXERCISING, start with six reps using the starting weight; when six becomes easy, increase the number of reps to eight, and then to ten. When ten becomes easy, increase the weight by two or three pounds and start over with six reps.

ONCE YOU HAVE MASTERED the basic moves and have begun to build strength, you may want to fine-tune your strengthening program to achieve specific goals:

TO DEVELOP MUSCLE POWER, do three to four sets of six reps, using the heaviest weight you can manage. The sets should have no more than a thirty- to forty-second rest between them. Schedule three to four workouts per week.

TO INCREASE MUSCLE SIZE, do four to five sets of eight to twelve reps, five or six days a week. Choose a weight that will allow you to complete at least eight repetitions using good form.

TO ENHANCE ENDURANCE, do two sets of fifteen to forty reps, using relatively light weights, performing each repetition slowly. Try to fit in ten to fourteen workouts per week (once in the morning, once in the evening).

The Importance of Being Aerobic

Aerobic exercise strengthens the cardiovascular system: the heart muscle literally becomes stronger, just like any other muscle that gets exercised, so that it can pump larger volumes of blood to muscles at a time, supplying them with the oxygen they need to work. (By the same token, like other muscles, the heart will atrophy with disuse.) Aerobic exercise also burns calories and fat, so you'll begin to look leaner and feel lighter. My classes are based on an hour of steady, nonstop movement, meaning that you get a good aerobic workout. But if you'd like to incorporate more cardiovascular work into your weekly routine, you have dozens of activities to choose from. Pick what's fun for you, and feel free to indulge in several, doing them on different days, depending on the weather and your mood and even where you are: if you're traveling, pack a jump rope, in-line skates, running shoes, swimsuit—and use them!

WHATEVER ACTIVITY YOU DO—cycle, swim, run on a track or treadmill, or in-line skate—start slowly, so that the muscles you'll be using have a chance to warm up for the specific activity. In other words, don't start running at full speed, but begin with fast walking or an easy jog. Do this for three to five minutes.

NOW GRADUALLY SPEED UP until you reach your training range, the intensity at which aerobic exercise will give you the most benefits. The best indicator of training range is your heart rate, expressed in beats per minute. The simplest way to determine target heart rate is to subtract your age from 220 and multiply the result by .70 for the low end of the range, and then by .85 for the high end of the range. For instance, if you're 25 years old, you'd do the math this way: 220 minus 25 is 195. Multiply that by .70 and you get 138.50; by .85, and you get 165.75. So your training range would be between 139 and 166 beats per minute. As you exercise, monitor your heart rate by taking your pulse: count the number of times your heart beats for ten seconds, then multiply by six to make sure you're working in your range. Take note of how you feel when you're exercising on target—how winded you feel, how sweaty you are. Pretty soon you'll be able to tell you're on target without going to the trouble of pulse counting.

YOU SHOULD KEEP GOING in training range for twenty to thirty minutes, then gradually slow down. Do not stop abruptly; spend two or three minutes moving at about the same pace you used when warming up.

The Fitness Five

Some health and fitness experts will tell you that there are three key elements of fitness—namely, cardiovascular health (or endurance), muscle strength, and flexibility—and that you have to develop and improve all three in order to be totally fit. This approach is fine if you are concerned only about strengthening your heart, losing weight, and otherwise improving your health. But if you want to enhance the quality of everyday living and/or improve your performance in sports, you also need to work on speed, and balance and coordination. What's more, I don't think there's a training method out there that is well rounded enough to develop all the physical qualities. The only way to cover every fitness base is to do more than one type of activity—a tactic that can be time-consuming, inconvenient, and expensive. Or you can adopt the Radu method: during the running sequence in the basic Class, switch directions, change

the footwork, even run backward—all of which helps to improve balance and coordination. Note that some of the simpler weight training moves are meant to be performed quickly: this develops speed.

You may be asking yourself why you should be worrying about how quickly you can lift a dumbbell, or how light you are on your feet. If you're really new to exercise, you may even be wondering why it matters if you can touch your toes or be able to run without stopping for twenty minutes. So that you won't think some of the things I advocate that you do in the name of fitness are crazy, here's a quick look at the five physical qualities and how improving them translates to easier work and more fun play.

strength

The ability to lift, push, pull, or move a weight or any external resistance through muscular contraction. This depends on the number of fibers in a given muscle, as well as their thickness. When you train you ask your muscle fibers to work, which "wakes up" the fibers that haven't been called upon before. Once they're put to work, they literally become larger—meaning more and bigger muscles are working. Before you can fully develop any of the other physical qualities, you have to work on strength.

Muscle strength is the foundation upon which you can build the other physical qualities, and therefore it is the most important. You need it for lifting and lugging anything, from a weighted barbell to a stack of books to a chubby toddler. The stronger you are, the more likely you are to perform well at all sports activities—rowing and swimming

hysical Qualities Defined

(where you have to work against the resistance of the water), racquet sports (the more power you get behind a serve or return, the faster it will whiz by your opponent), and so on.

speed

The ability to execute a single movement or a complex exercise within a specific period of time, or cover a distance in the shortest time. There are two types: speed of reaction (response to an external stimulus) and speed of execution (how many times you can hit a punching bag in a specific amount of time or how fast you can run a certain distance, for example). Speed of execution is based on strength. Speed is needed in track-and-field events such as sprinting (up to 400 meters) and long jumping; speed swimming; speed skating; fast bicycling; fencing; boxing—any sport that requires a quick reaction time, like tennis, basketball, baseball, and soccer.

endurance

The ability to sustain an activity for a long time. There are three aspects of endurance: the lungs' capacity to take in large amounts of oxygen to be passed on to the bloodstream; the heart's ability to pump ample amounts of oxygen-rich blood to working muscles; and muscles' ability to work for a sustained period of time without fatiguing. Any aerobic sport—such as running, power walking, bicycling, cross-country skiing, kayaking, swimming, hiking, jumping rope, and ice or in-line skating—as well as fast-paced activities like tennis and boxing, requires endurance. If you're physically fatigued, your ability to make decisions or do any sort of brain work will be compromised.

flexibility

The ability of a joint to move through a full range of motion, depending on the elasticity of the mus-cle and connective tissue that surround the joint. The same activities that improve flexibility, such as yoga, dance, and gymnastics, need it. Flexibility also comes into play whenever we have to reach up for something, like a book on a shelf, or stretch down to tie a shoelace. Flexibility contributes to agility (the stiffer you are, the less coordinated you are) and strength (the longer a muscle is, the more powerful it is; a flexible muscle is a young muscle).

balance and coordination

These abilities integrate your nervous system with the other physical qualities. Good balance and coordination allow you to visualize a movement and physically carry it out. Just about everything you do requires coordination and agility, from hiking and swimming to sports in which you have to be ready to move in any direction at any time, like tennis, basketball, or boxing.

The Class

Candice Bergen once commented about my Class, "The good news is that it's only an hour." Candice claimed she couldn't make it down the stairs after her first workout at my gym, but that didn't stop her from bringing in friends, and she began training with me privately. She became so dedicated to her workouts, and achieved such stunning results—strong and lean, with beautiful muscle definition—that when she autographed a copy of her 1984 book *Knock Wood* for me, she signed it Candina Schwarzenegger! The chances are good that you won't be able to make it down the stairs after you complete the workout in this chapter either. The Class comprises the exercises that are fundamental to my program; these are the simplest of moves, but I've put them together into a conditioning program that will hit on every single muscle—muscles you didn't know you had.

But once you've perfected the moves in this routine, you will have laid a solid, all-around fitness foundation that will keep you primed for just about any physical challenge life throws your way—from rearranging furniture to training for a marathon. This is a total conditioning program that will develop all the physical qualities—strength, speed, endurance, and flexibility, plus balance and coordination—you need to become not only fit but agile, graceful, and confident in all that you do. This is the routine that will put you at the 80 percent of physical potential that's essential to living life fully. It's the type of workout that John Kennedy relies on between training for intense activities; in fact I urge all my students, famous or not, to take a class two or three times a week.

Before you start, turn on your answering machine, turn off your TV, and get yourself to a place where you can have total privacy for at least an hour. You don't want any distractions; you need to concentrate on what your body is doing and feeling every step of the way, or you'll just be going through the motions. This isn't the time to half-heartedly pump a dumbbell up and down while you have one eye on the evening news. Do each move with purpose and conviction, and move the body part you're working through its full range of motion. When you lunge or jump, engage the entire ankle-knee-hip chain, which absorbs shocks and therefore will not put unnecessary strain on your back. Shorten the move, and you short-change the benefits. Whenever you can, place a hand on the muscle you're working to get an idea of how it functions. The more familiar you are with the way your body works, the more efficiently you will be able to train and use it.

Another word to the wise: Don't skip the warm-up! This portion of the workout may seem easy, but in fact it is probably the most important part of the entire routine. You can't just jump right in and expect your body and mind to be ready for heavy-duty activity; you need to ease each aspect into gear, like warming up a car. As you do the warm-up, you move your joints; in order to move them, muscles must contract. Those muscles need oxygenated blood to contract, so the heart and lungs must become involved. (If you plan to do an aerobic activity like running or cycling, you should always do a general warm-up and then the warm-up that's specific to the activity.) Your temperature rises; this literally warms up the muscles so that they're more pliable. And as you begin to concentrate on moving your body, your mind becomes focused on what you're doing, so that you're not only physically ready for exercise but mentally and emotionally primed as well. To do this most efficiently, you'll go from slow to fast movements, from short-range movements to wider-range movements, and you'll work systematically from the upper body, which consists of smaller muscles, to the lower body, which is made up of larger muscles.

One more thing: push yourself as hard as you can, but pay attention to how you're feeling. There's no reason to get hurt doing this workout. You can tell the difference between taking your physical abilities to the limit and just a little beyond—that's how you'll make progress—and overdoing it to the point of injury. If you become so winded that you can't catch your breath or talk, slow down. If when you're doing a move, you become so fatigued that you lose good form or can't get through a full range of motion, then stop that exercise, rest, and then move on. Otherwise, grit your teeth and tough it out. Now let's get to work!

Training is a rehearsal for life.

The Class

WARM UP

NECK
Consult a doctor if you experience prolonged dizziness.

1.
Stand with feet shoulder-width apart. Look up and down.
Reps: 6–10 each way
Sets: 1
Weights: None

2.
Look over each shoulder side to side.
Reps: 6–10 each way
Sets: 1
Weights: None

3.
Bring your ear to your left shoulder, then to your right.
Reps: 6–10 each way
Sets: 1
Weights: None

SHOULDERS
4.
Scissors
Swing left arm by your ear and right arm by your side, alternating arms continuously.
Reps: 6–10 each way
Sets: 1
Weights: None

5.
Crossovers
Cross your arms in front of your chest and swing them back out to sides, arms slightly bent and parallel to the floor.
Reps: 6–10 each way
Sets: 1
Weights: None

6.
Double arm rotations
Extend both arms out to the side, elbows slightly bent, in a relaxed position. Circle both arms forward; then circle them back.
Reps: 6–10 each way
Sets: 1
Weights: None

WAIST

7.

Side bends

Widen your stance slightly and bend at the waist to the right, keeping your lower body stable and bringing your left arm overhead. Switch directions and continue alternating right and left. Do not hold position; move continuously.

Reps: 6–10 each way
Sets: 1
Weights: None

8.

Waist twists

Cross arms in front of chest and grasp hands, keeping arms parallel to ground; twist right and left at waist continuously.

Reps: 6–10 each way
Sets: 1
Weights: None

9.

Back extensions

Standing with feet shoulder-width apart and knees slightly bent, bend your torso toward your toes, allowing your arms to relax down toward the floor. Stand up tall, reaching your arms toward the ceiling, then bend forward and down again in a continuous movement.

Reps: 4–10
Sets: 1
Weights: None

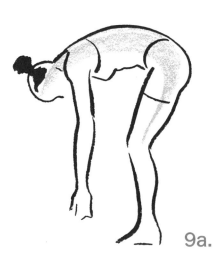

9a.

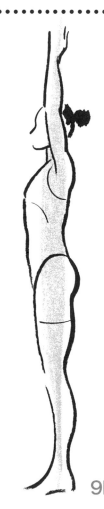

9b.

10.
Torso circles
Stand with feet shoulder-width apart, toes forward, knees relaxed. Place hands on hips, bend forward slightly at the waist, then move torso right, back, and left, making a full circle. Repeat all reps before changing direction.
Reps: 6–10 each way
Sets: 1
Weights: None

11.
Windmills
Stand, bending at waist, and touch right foot with left hand, then left foot with right hand, constantly swinging your arms to each foot. Your head and shoulders should follow the movement of the upper arm in order to increase range of motion.
Reps: 6–10 each way
Sets: 1
Weights: None

HIPS/KNEES
12.
Partial side lunges
Stand with feet slightly wider than shoulder-width apart, toes pointing forward, hands on knees. Keep your hip area tight and your shoulders relaxed. Bend your right leg and straighten your left, allowing the toes of your left foot to come off the floor; make sure that your right knee does not extend past your toes. Repeat on the other side, and continue alternating from right to left.
Reps: 6–10 each way .
Sets: 1
Weights: None

13.
Deep side lunges
Widen stance and bend knees for deep side lunges to stretch inner thigh. Remain in deep lunge position and pulse slightly on each leg, then move on to lunge twists.
Reps: 6–10 each way
Sets: 1
Weights: None

14.
Lunge twists
Stand with your right knee bent, your left leg extended straight behind you, toes on floor. Place your hands on your hips. Jump lightly and turn in the air so that you land with your left knee bent and your right leg extended behind you. Continue jumping and twisting without pausing. After completing all reps of lunge twists, bring feet closer together and twist hips, hopping continuously.
Reps: 12–20 each way
Sets: 1
Weights: None

15.
Front lunges
Step forward with your left leg, keeping the knee bent slightly without stretching all the way to the floor; do not allow your left knee to extend past your toes. Let your right leg straighten naturally, with as wide a stance as possible for stretching hamstrings. Switch.
Reps: 6–10 each way
Sets: 1
Weights: None

EXERCISES

FOUR-WAY SQUATS

Complete three rotations with legs together, one leg forward, one leg to side, and one leg to back. Do light jumps for 20–30 seconds after each rotation.

16.

Legs together

Squat, feet together and both hands on floor a few inches in front of toes. Straighten both legs, keeping your hands on the floor (or as close as possible). Squat up and down in a controlled, unbroken movement.

Reps: beginning 6
        intermediate 8
        advanced 10
Sets: 3
Weights: None

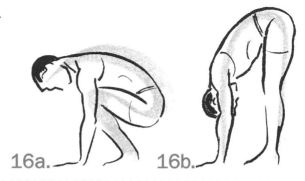

16a. 16b.

17.

One leg forward

Squat, feet together and both hands on floor a few inches in front of toes. Stand, bringing your right leg straight in front of you and parallel to the floor, and raise both arms overhead. Return to first position, then lift your left leg. Continue, alternating legs.

Reps: beginning 6
        intermediate 8
        advanced 10
Sets: 3
Weights: None

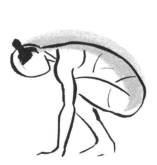

17a.

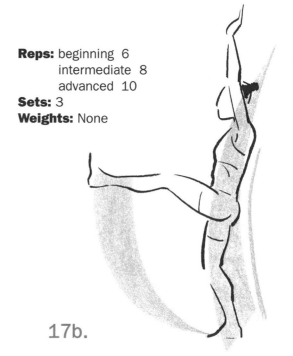

17b.

18.

One leg to side

Squat, feet together and both hands on floor a few inches in front of toes. Stand up, bring both arms overhead and your right leg straight out to the side so that it is parallel to the floor. Return to start, and lift your left leg to the side. Continue, alternating legs.

Reps: beginning 6
intermediate 8
advanced 10

Sets: 3
Weights: None

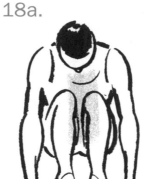

18a.

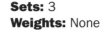

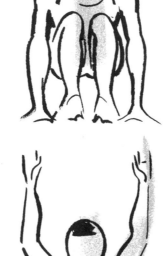

18b.

19.

One leg to back

Assume same position as previous squat, standing and bringing your right leg straight behind you. Return to start, and lift your left leg behind you. Continue, alternating legs.

Reps: beginning 6
intermediate 8
advanced 10

Sets: 3
Weights: None

LUNGES
20.

Front lunges

Stand, arms bent at waist level. Lift your left leg, knee bent 90 degrees and thigh parallel to floor. Step far forward with your left leg, extending leg and lowering your body toward the floor; do not allow your left knee to extend past your toes. Let your right leg straighten naturally, but firmly. Push back and up from your left toe to your heel, bringing your knee up to return to starting position.

Reps: beginning 6
intermediate 8
advanced 10

Sets: 3
Weights: None

21.
Reverse lunges
Step back, extending left leg behind you. Lower your body toward the floor and reach your left leg as far back as it can go, then push up to starting position. The right knee should not extend past your toes. Complete 1 set on left leg, 1 set on right, then rest 10 to 15 seconds before starting with left leg again.

Reps: beginning 6
 intermediate 8
 advanced 10
Sets: 3
Weights: None

RUNNING
For confined area. If you have the space, jog around in circles or on a path. Repeat entire sequence once, 10–20 seconds for each running exercise.

22.
a. Run in place at a relaxed pace, elbows bent 90 degrees, hands loosely fisted.
b. Knees up: Pick up the pace, bringing your knees up toward your chest and moving your arms back and forth from the shoulder like pistons.
c. Run in place.
d. Heels back: Bring your heels to your buttocks and pump your arms.
e. Run in place (rest time).
f. Lightly jump up and down on both feet.
g. Run in place (rest time).
h. Knees up.
i. Run in place.
j. Heels back.
k. Run in place.
l. Scissor your legs forward and back continuously in small lunges.
m. Run in place (rest time).
n. Knees up.

o. Run in place.
p. Heels back.
q. Run in place.
r. Jump lightly and twist your hips continuously.
Reps: repeat entire sequence once
Sets: 1
Weights: None

ARMS
23.
Push-ups
Standard: Place your hands on the floor about shoulder-width apart, fingers pointing forward. Extend your legs behind you, feet together and balanced on toes. Make sure your head is in line with your spine. Tighten your abs and tuck your pelvis so that your body is straight. Keeping your body stiff as a board, bend your elbows until your chest is almost touching the floor, then return to starting position.
Modified: Kneel on hands and knees, hands shoulder-width apart, fingers facing forward. Bring your feet off the floor, tuck your pelvis, and tighten your knees. Bend your elbows until your chest is just a few inches from the floor, then return to starting position. Rest 15–20 seconds after all three sets.

Reps: beginning 6
 intermediate 8
 advanced 10
Sets: 3
Weights: None

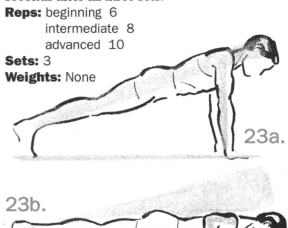

23a.

23b.

WEIGHTS
Complete three rotations of bench presses, lateral flyes, pullovers, and big circles, resting for 30 seconds after each rotation.

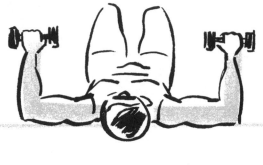

24a.

24.

Bench presses

Lie on your back, knees bent, holding a dumbbell in each hand. Extend both arms toward the ceiling, palms facing forward. Bring elbows toward the floor, then straighten arms back toward ceiling.

Reps: beginning 15
intermediate 20
advanced 25
Sets: 3
Weights: 5; 8; 10 lbs.

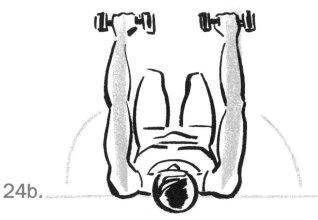

24b.

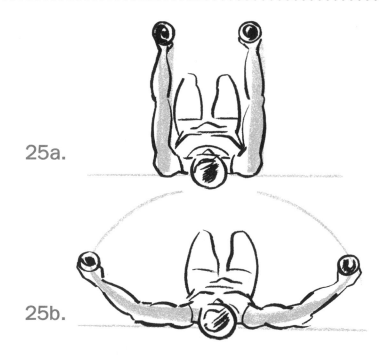

25a.

25b.

25.

Lateral flyes

Lie on your back, knees bent, holding a dumbbell in each hand, arms extended toward the ceiling, palms facing in and elbows slightly bent. Inhaling, open both arms wide to the sides as far as you can, feeling a stretch across your chest. Exhale and return to starting position, squeezing your chest as you bring the dumbbells together.

Reps: beginning 15
intermediate 20
advanced 25
Sets: 3
Weights: 3; 5 lbs.

26.

Pullovers

Lie on your back. Hold a
dumbbell in each hand,
knuckles facing in and close
together, elbows slightly
bent. Inhaling, bring both
arms over your head as
far as you can, tapping the
weights lightly on the floor,
then exhale and bring them
back to starting position.
Reps: 15
Sets: 3
Weights: 10; 16; 20 lbs.

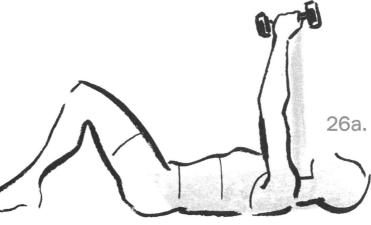

26a.

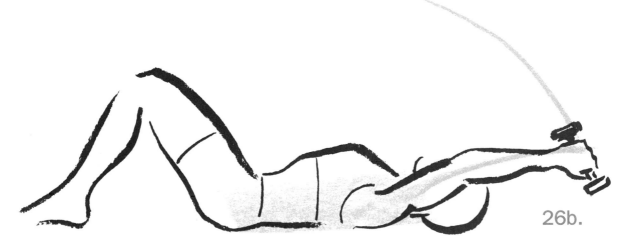

26b.

27.

Big circles, in and out

Put weights aside. Lie on
back, knees bent, and bring
your arms straight over your
chest. Circle arms to the
side, overhead, down in
front of you, and out to sides
again; reverse directions
after six reps.

Reps: 6 each way
Sets: 3
Weights: None

Complete three rotations of curls, overhead presses, lateral raises, bent-over rows, and side bends, resting for 30 seconds after each rotation.

28.

Standing biceps curls

Stand, feet shoulder-width apart, knees slightly bent. Grasp a dumbbell in each hand and hold your arms at your sides, palms facing upward and elbows at your sides. Keeping your upper arms pressed against your sides, exhale and bend your arms to bring the weights to your shoulders. Inhale and return to starting position.

Reps: beginning 6
intermediate 8
advanced 10

Sets: 3

Weights: Women 3–5 lbs.
Men 8–12 lbs.

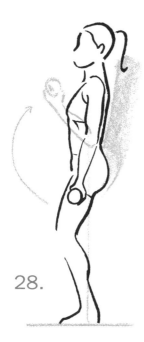

28.

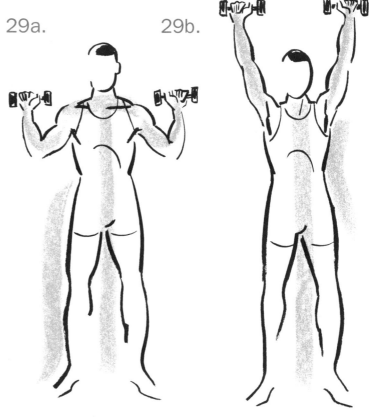

29a.   29b.

29.

Overhead presses

Stand with your feet shoulder-width apart, knees slightly bent. Hold a dumbbell in each hand at shoulder level, fingers facing forward, elbows pointing down. Exhale and press both weights straight up toward the ceiling, keeping them even. Inhale and bring them back to starting position.

Reps: beginning 6
intermediate 8
advanced 10

Sets: 3

Weights: Women 3–5 lbs.
Men 8–12 lbs.

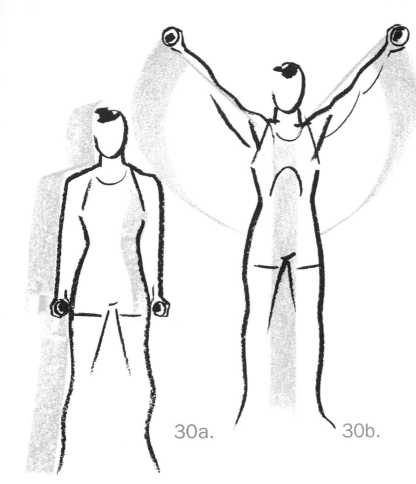

30a. **30b.**

30.

Lateral raises

Stand, feet shoulder-width apart, arms at sides, elbows slightly bent, and a dumbbell in each hand. Knees are slightly bent. Raise both arms straight out to sides as high as is comfortable; keep your shoulders pressed down—do not squeeze them toward ears.

Reps: beginning 6
intermediate 8
advanced 10

Sets: 3

Weights: Women 3–5 lbs.
Men 8–12 lbs.

31.

Bent-over rows

Holding a dumbbell in each hand, bend forward and extend both arms toward the floor, palms facing your shins. Bend your elbows toward the ceiling to bring the weights to chest level.

Reps: beginning 6
intermediate 8
advanced 10

Sets: 3

Weights: Women 3–5 lbs.
Men 8–12 lbs.

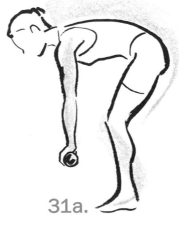

31a.

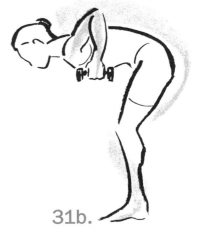

31b.

32.

Side bends

Stand, feet slightly more than shoulder-width apart, knees slightly bent. Hold a dumbbell in each hand, arms at sides. Bend your torso to the left, bringing your right elbow toward the ceiling, then return to start. Finish reps on right side before starting on left side.

Reps: 10 each way
Sets: 1
Weights: Women 3–5 lbs.
Men 8–12 lbs.

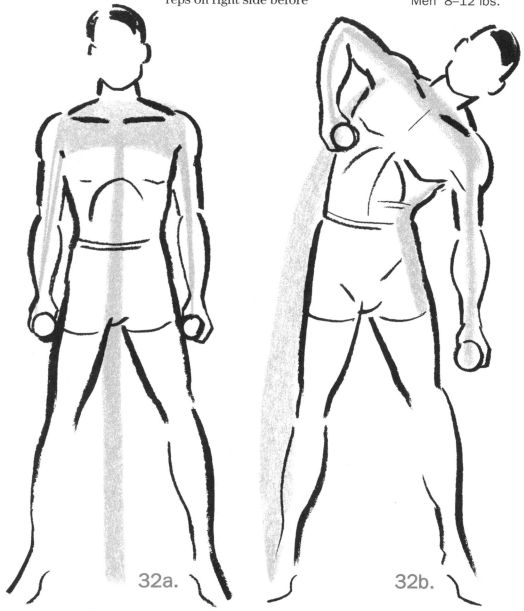

32a.

32b.

Complete three rotations of reverse curls, overhead presses, front raises, bent-over rows, and side bends, resting for 30 seconds after each rotation.

33.
Reverse curls

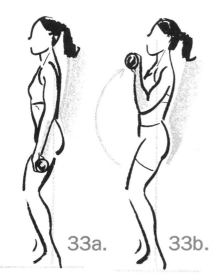

33a.   33b.

Stand, feet shoulder-width apart, knees slightly bent. Grasp a dumbbell in each hand and hold your arms at your sides, palms facing downward and elbows at your sides. Keeping your upper arms pressed against your sides, exhale and bend your arms to bring the weights to your shoulders. Inhale and return to starting position.

Reps: beginning 6
intermediate 8
advanced 10

Sets: 3

Weights: Women 3–5 lbs.
Men 8–12 lbs.

34.
Overhead presses

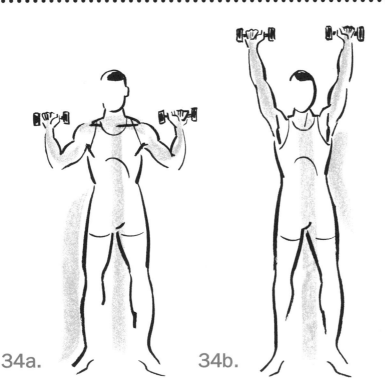

34a.   34b.

Stand with your feet shoulder-width apart, knees slightly bent. Hold a dumbbell in each hand at shoulder level, fingers facing forward, elbows pointing down. Exhale and press both weights straight up toward the ceiling, keeping them even. Inhale and bring them back to starting position.

Reps: beginning 6
intermediate 8
advanced 10

Sets: 3

Weights: Women 3–5 lbs.
Men 8–12 lbs.

35.

Front raises

Stand with feet about shoulder-width apart, knees relaxed, a dumbbell in each hand, resting on thighs. Elbows should be slightly bent. Raise both arms toward the ceiling until at eye level.

Reps: beginning 6
intermediate 8
advanced 10

Sets: 3

Weights: Women 3–5 lbs.
Men 8–12 lbs.

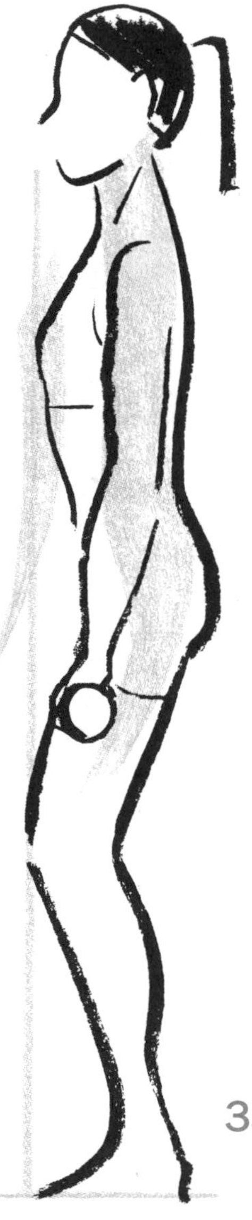

35a.

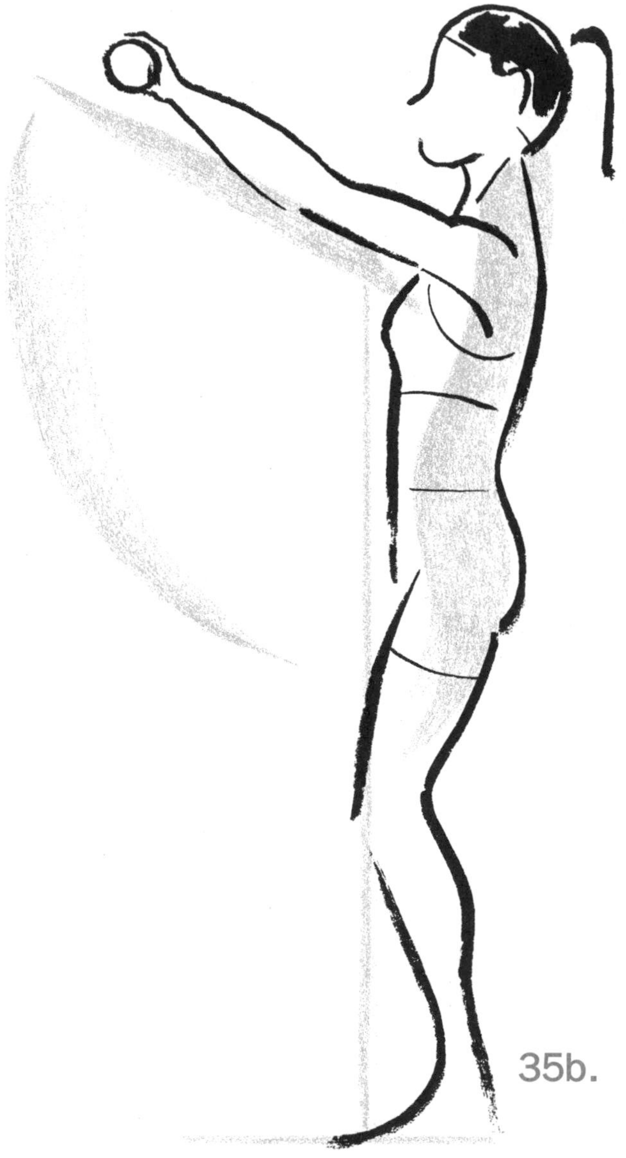

35b.

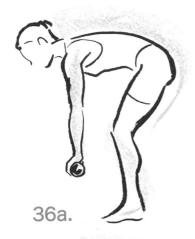

36a.

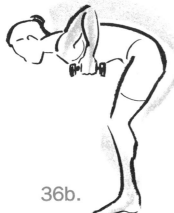

36b.

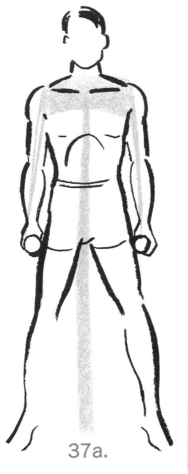

37a.

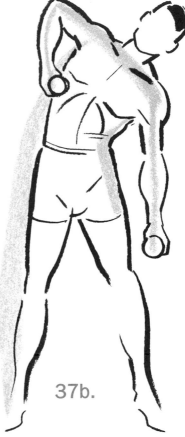

37b.

36.

Bent-over rows

Holding a dumbbell in each hand, bend forward and extend both arms toward the floor, palms facing your shins, knees slightly bent. Bend your elbows toward the ceiling to bring the weights to chest level.

Reps: beginning 6
intermediate 8
advanced 10

Sets: 3

Weights: Women 3–5 lbs.
Men 8–12 lbs.

37.

Side bends

Stand, feet slightly more than shoulder-width apart, knees slightly bent. Hold a dumbbell in each hand, arms at sides. Bend your torso to the left, bringing your right elbow toward the ceiling, then return to start. Finish reps on right side before starting on left side.

Reps: 10 each way

Sets: 1

Weights: Women 3–5 lbs.
Men 8–12 lbs.

Complete three rotations of curls, behind-the-neck barbell presses, lateral raises, bent-over rows, and side bends, resting for 30 seconds after each rotation.

38.

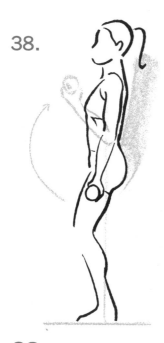

39a. 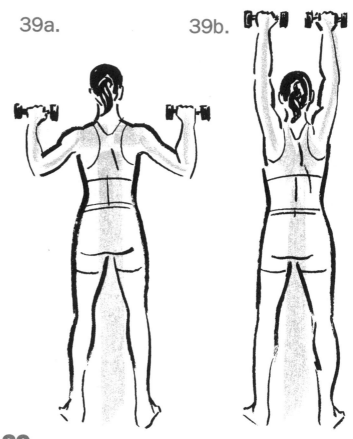 39b.

38.
Standing biceps curls
Stand, feet shoulder-width apart, knees slightly bent. Grasp a dumbbell in each hand and hold your arms at your sides, palms facing upward and elbows at your sides. Keeping your upper arms pressed against your sides, exhale and bend your arms to bring the weights to your shoulders. Inhale and return to starting position.

Reps: beginning 6
      intermediate 8
      advanced 10
Sets: 3
Weights: Women 3–5 lbs.
      Men 8–12 lbs.

39.
Behind-the-neck barbell presses
Stand with feet shoulder-width apart, knees slightly bent. Hold a dumbbell in each hand, slightly above and behind shoulders. Press both arms toward ceiling, then return to start.

Reps: beginning 6
      intermediate 8
      advanced 10
Sets: 3
Weights: Women 3–5 lbs.
      Men 8–12 lbs.

40.

Lateral raises

Stand, feet shoulder-width apart, arms at sides, a dumbbell in each hand. Knees are slightly bent. Raise both arms straight out to sides as high as is comfortable; keep your shoulders pressed down—do not squeeze them toward ears.

Reps: beginning 6
intermediate 8
advanced 10
Sets: 3
Weights: Women 3–5 lbs.
Men 8–12 lbs.

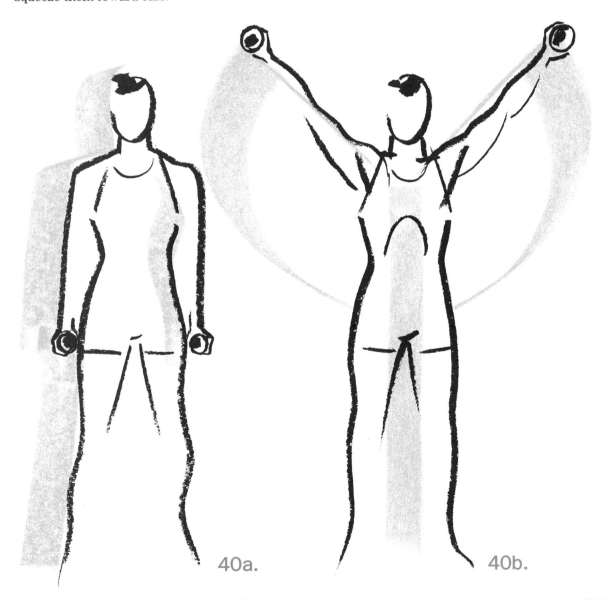

40a.   40b.

41.

Bent-over rows
Holding a dumbbell in each hand, bend forward and extend both arms toward the floor, palms facing your shins, knees slightly bent. Bend your elbows toward the ceiling to bring the weights to chest level.

Reps: beginning 6
intermediate 8
advanced 10

Sets: 3

Weights: Women 3–5 lbs.
Men 8–12 lbs.

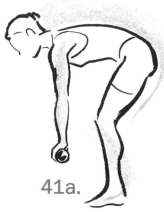

41a.

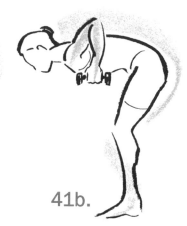

41b.

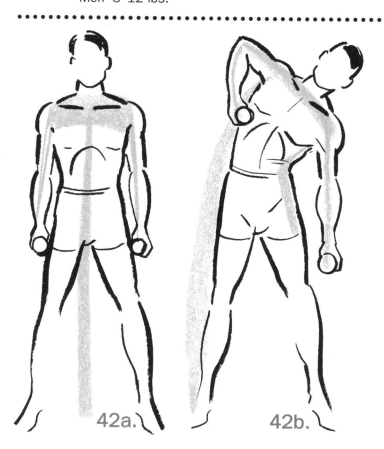

42a.

42b.

42.

Side bends
Stand, feet slightly more than shoulder-width apart, knees slightly bent. Hold a dumbbell in each hand, arms at sides. Bend your torso to the left, bringing your right elbow toward the ceiling, then return to start. Finish reps on right side before starting on left side.

Reps: 10 each way

Sets: 1

Weights: Women 3–5 lbs.
Men 8–12 lbs.

WAIST

Caution: If you have any back problems, continue with 2–3 extra sets of crunches and forgo the sit-ups and leg lifts. Aim for a total of 200–300 reps in abdominal exercises. After reverse leg curls and again after tuck jackknives, stretch the full length of your body while still on your back. Bring your knees to your chest and wrap your arms around your shins, chin to chest; rock back and forth 4 to 10 times.

43.

Crunches

Lie on your back, legs bent and raised, ankles crossed. Place your hands behind your head, elbows extended, and press your lower back into the floor. Lift your shoulders and buttocks up, bringing your elbows and knees together and contracting your abdominals.

Reps: 25
Sets: 1
Weights: None

44.

Side crunches

Similar to a crunch, but instead lift your shoulders and buttocks up, squeezing your left side and bringing your left elbow and left knee together. Switch to right side after completion of set.

Reps: 25 left side, then 25 right side
Sets: 1
Weights: None

45.

Reverse leg curls

Similar to a crunch, but instead keep your shoulders against the floor while bringing your knees to your chest. Touch heels to floor each rep, keeping your lower back pressed against the floor.

Reps: 25
Sets: 1
Weights: None

46.

Sit-ups

Lie on your back, knees bent, feet apart. Bend your elbows close to your sides, hands fisted. Sit up, straightening your arms past your legs.

Reps: beginning 10
intermediate 15
advanced 25
Sets: 1
Weights: None

46a.

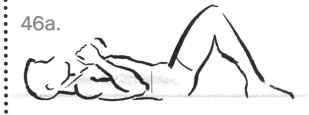

46b.

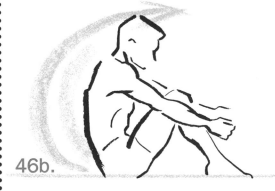

r back with arms by your sides,
your head on the floor. Bend your
legs ghtly, feet together and heels on the
floor. Pressing your lower back into the
floor, raise both legs toward the ceiling as
high as you can before slowly lowering
them to starting position. Try not to touch

the floor with your feet on successive lifts.
If needed, place pillow under head.

Reps: beginning 10
intermediate 15
advanced 25

Sets: 1
Weights: None

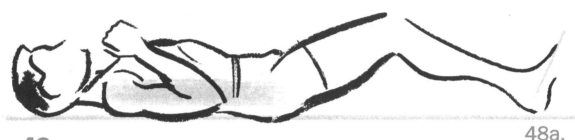

48a.

48.

Tuck jackknives

Lie on your back, arms bent at sides, hands
fisted. Bend your legs slightly, feet together
and heels on the floor. Sit up, letting arms
extend forward as necessary and bringing
both knees to your chest. Return to start
slowly, holding your abdominals tight as
you lower your torso and legs.

Reps: beginning 10
intermediate 15
advanced 25

Sets: 1
Weights: None

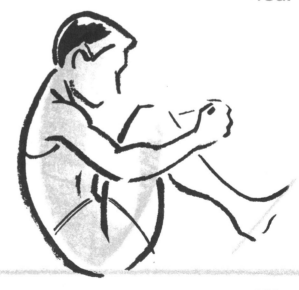

48b.

COOL DOWN

49.
Arches

Lie on your stomach, arms extended straight above your head, legs together. Raise your arms and legs simultaneously, hold for a second, and then lower both to the floor slowly.

Reps: beginning 6
intermediate 8
advanced 10

Sets: 1

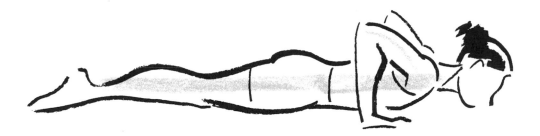

50.
Cobras

Lie on your stomach, legs together, arms bent, and hands at chest level. Straighten both arms and lift your torso and abdomen off the floor. Hold for 3 seconds, then return to start. If this causes any back pain, allow arms to bend or discontinue this move.

Reps: beginning 6
intermediate 8
advanced 10

Sets: 1

50a.

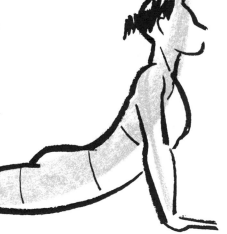

50b.

STRETCHES
Hold each for 10 seconds, or count to 12.

51.
Diamond

Sit up straight and bring your feet toward you, soles together. Use your hands to gently pull your feet closer, pressing down with your knees so that you feel a stretch all along your inner thighs.

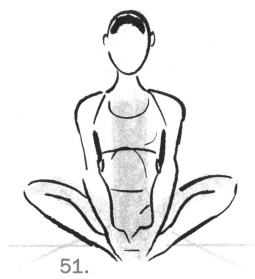

51.

52.
Straddle

Sit up straight, legs as wide apart as is comfortable, feet flexed. Raise both arms overhead. Stretch forward at the hips as far as you can. Don't worry if you can only go a few inches; the point is to feel a stretch along your inner thighs. Stretch to left toe; to right toe; to middle.

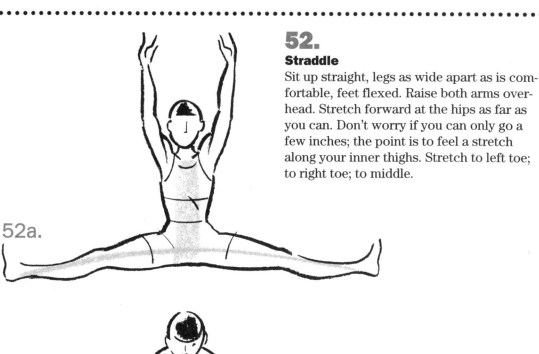

52a.

52b.

53.
Pretzel

Sit up straight with your left leg extended in front of you, your hands relaxed by your sides. Bend your right leg and cross it over the left, setting your right foot flat on the floor beside your left knee. Twist to the right, bringing your left arm outside of your right knee; use your left arm as leverage against your right leg to help you twist further. Then switch sides.

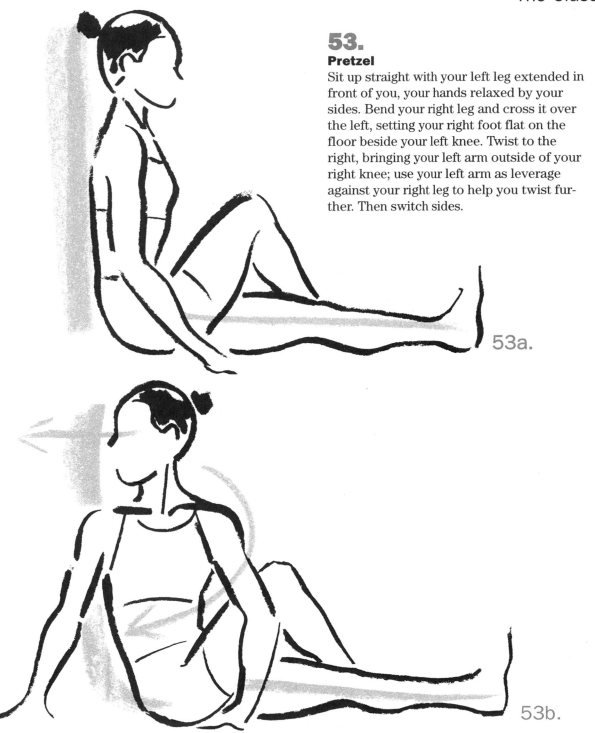

53a.

53b.

The Time-Efficient Program

What's the number-one reason people give for skimping on exercise? Too few hours in the day. Thinking that exercise is a time-consuming obligation requiring at least an hour and a half to be worth it, you may throw up your hands in despair. Where can I spare ninety minutes in my schedule? Some people rank fitness as a luxury, placing it far down on their list of priorities, even though in reality, regular activity is as crucial to life as eating, drinking, breathing, and sleeping. The stamina and energy earned from it actually make it *easier* to complete even the most mundane tasks more efficiently.

In fact, exercise doesn't have to be laborious, exact, and performance-oriented all the time. There's plenty you can do in a hotel room or even in your office to maintain not only your fitness level but also the habit of exercising. For those days when you really don't have a full hour to do the Class, here's a pared-down version that requires no equipment—not so much as a dumbbell. (You will need a sturdy chair that can be positioned with its back against a wall for stability.) I've divided the routine into three sections—warm-up, main exercises, and cool-down. Do the first and last sections once each and repeat the main exercises one, two, or three times, depending on how much time you have.

WARM UP

1.
Breathe in deeply, bringing both arms out to the side and then up to the ceiling; exhale as you lower your arms back to your sides.
Reps: 6–10 each side

2.
Bring your ear to your left shoulder, then to your right.
Reps: 6–10 each side

3.
Look left over shoulder, then right over shoulder.
Reps: 6–10 each side

4.
Extend both arms out to the side, elbows slightly bent, in a relaxed position. Circle both arms forward; then circle them back.
Reps: 6–10 each way

5.
Bend at the waist to the right, keeping your lower body stable and bringing your left arm overhead; switch directions and continue alternating.
Reps: 6–10 each side

6.
Clasp your hands in front of your chest, elbows up, and twist your torso to the right, and then to the left.
Reps: 6–10

7.
Stand with your legs comfortably apart and your arms extended forward at shoulder level and slightly angled outward (forming a "V"): Lift your right foot to touch your left hand (without dropping your left arm); repeat on the other side.
Reps: 6–10 each side

8.
Still standing, place your hands behind your neck and bring your right elbow to your left knee and your knee to your elbow, meeting in the middle; repeat on the other side.
Reps: 6–10 each side

9.
Walk in place, elbows bent 90 degrees, bringing just your heels off the ground.
Time in seconds: 10–20

10.
Continue walking, raising your knees all the way up.
Time in seconds: 10–20

11.
Continue walking, lifting your heels toward your butt.
Time in seconds: 10–20

12.
Stand with your head bowed and hands on bent knees. Then elevate yourself: lift your heels so you're on the balls of your feet, straighten your knees, and raise your hands high.
Time in seconds: 10–20

EXERCISES

Start with lower amount of time and reps and build up slowly.

13.
Running sequence

Complete three rotations of the four running exercises that follow, each exercise lasting 10–20 seconds. Lightly run in place for 10–20 seconds after each rotation.
• Run in place, knees up
• Run in place, heels back
• Jump on both feet, bending your knees slightly as you land and raising both arms as if shooting a basketball

14.
Chair squats

Stand in front of a sturdy chair with your hands on your thighs; squat until you're almost sitting on the chair, then return to starting position.
Reps: 6–25
Sets: 1–3
Rest time, in seconds: 20

15.
Triceps dip

Position the chair with its back legs against a wall. Stand with your back to the chair and reach behind you to place both hands on its seat, about shoulder-width apart. Bend your knees to a comfortable position and lower and raise your torso by bending and straightening your elbows.
Reps: 6–25

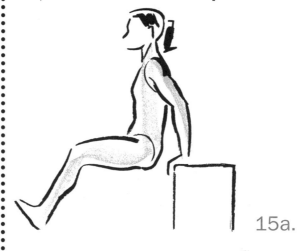

15a.

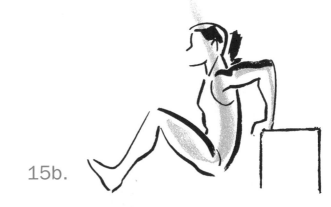

15b.

16.

All-purpose crunches

Lie on your back with your right leg bent and your right hand behind your head, your left leg straight and your left arm alongside your body. Keeping your lower back pressed into the floor, simultaneously lift your left knee and right elbow toward each other. Complete all the reps on one side before switching.

Reps: 6–25 each side

17.

Push-ups

Standard: Place your hands on the floor about shoulder-width apart, fingers pointing forward. Extend your legs behind you, feet together and balanced on toes. Make sure your head is in line with your spine. Tighten your abs and tuck your pelvis so that your body is straight. Keeping your body stiff as a board, bend your elbows until your chest is just a few inches from the floor, then return to starting position.

Modified: Kneel on hands and knees, hands shoulder-width apart, fingers facing forward. Bring your feet off the floor, tuck your pelvis, and tighten your knees. Bend your elbows until your chest is just a few inches from the floor, then return to starting position.

Reps: 6–25

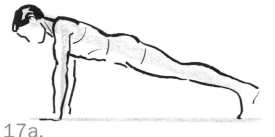

17a.

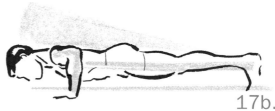

17b.

18.

Opposite arm and leg lift

Lie on your stomach with your legs straight and both arms extended overhead. Raise your left leg and right arm at the same time, then lower them. Do all reps on one side before switching to the other.

Reps: 4–10 each side

COOL DOWN

STRETCHES
Hold each stretch 10 seconds, or count to 12.

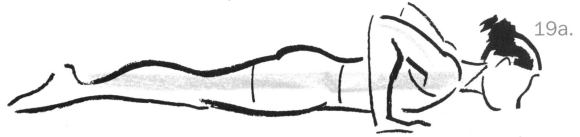

19a.

19.

Cobra
Lie on your stomach, legs together, arms bent, and hands at chest level. Straighten both arms and lift your torso and abdomen off the floor. Hold for a second, then return to start. If this causes any back pain, please discontinue this move. Then come up on your hands and knees and bring your torso back over your thighs, keeping your hands in place; hold.

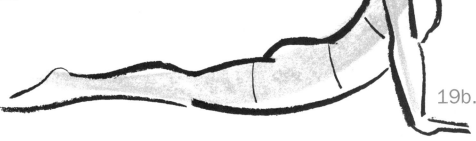

19b.

20.

Half-diamond
Sit up with your right leg extended at a slight angle, with your left leg bent so that your foot is tucked against your right upper thigh; stretch your torso over your right leg, reaching for your toes; hold, then switch legs.

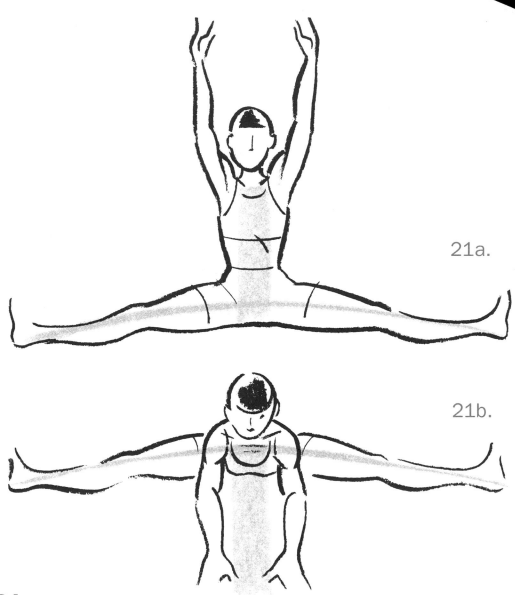

21a.

21b.

21.

Straddle

Extend both legs in a wide "V" and stretch
your torso over your right leg, and hold;
over your left leg, and hold; and then in
the middle.

...ur right leg extended in
...ands relaxed by your
...left leg and cross it over the
...your left foot flat on the floor
...right knee. Twist to the left,
b...g your right arm outside of your left
kne...use your right arm as leverage against
your left leg to help you twist further. Then,
starting with your left leg extended, repeat
stretch to opposite side. Remember throughout to keep your back straight.

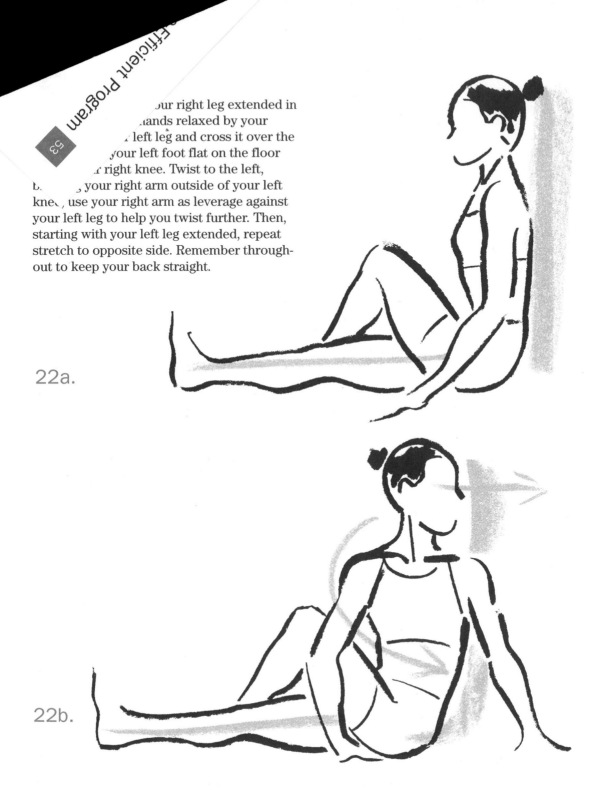

22a.

22b.

23.

"Rocking chair" back rolls

Bring your knees to your chest and wrap your arms around your shins, chin to chest; rock back and forth 4–10 times.

24.

Over-thigh stretch

Come onto hands and knees, stretch back over your thighs again; hold. Then return to hands and knees, curl your toes under, and straighten your legs, keeping your hands as close to the floor as you can; hold, then roll up to standing.

25.

Neck stretch

Wrap your right arm over your head so you can touch your left ear; gently pull your head to the right; hold and switch sides. Then place both hands behind your head and bring your chin to your chest; hold.

26.

Side stretch

Grab your left wrist with your right hand and stretch your left arm toward the ceiling and out to the right side; hold, then switch sides.

27.

Reverse shoulder stretch

Clasp your hands behind your back; bending your knees, bend forward at the hips. Keep your back straight and stretch your arms overhead.

28.

Doorjamb

Place your left palm against a doorjamb, left arm straight and parallel to the floor. Turn your body toward the right and away from the doorjamb so that you feel a stretch across the left side of your chest; hold, then switch sides.

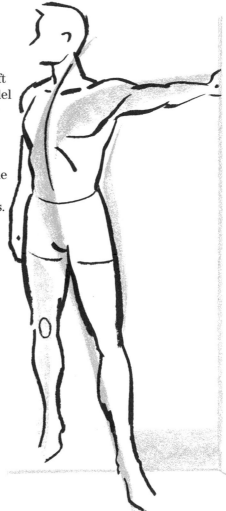

28.

Personal Training

As you know by now, my personal training is a very special experience in which I become a total fitness coach attuned to the individual's every need. This detailed application of my methods is what has attracted legions of famous students to me over the past two decades, as well as bringing countless people in search of the ultimate fitness program. For you to have some sense of the overall Radu experience, I want to try to give you some of the benefits of this intense one-on-one training here in this book.

In this chapter, I am going to share with you actual workouts that I devised for some of my best-known students, which you too can use in your own training. That flabby belly and pain-prone lower back will benefit greatly from Regis Philbin's abdominal and back strengthening routine. The flexibility and strength training that prepared Vanessa Williams for the title role in the play *Kiss of the Spider Woman* will come in handy for any parent whose day involves picking through a toy-strewn room and balancing a baby on one hip and a laundry basket on another while climbing the stairs thirty

times. And John Kennedy's adventure training is inspiring to anyone who wants to take their well-developed body into the outdoors, even if it's the park down the street instead of halfway across the globe.

As you will see, I always start by trying to re-create the challenge the student is preparing for inside the safe and controlled environment of the gym. A wonderful young woman named Sandy came to my gym a few years ago to rehabilitate a broken hand. Sandy is a real outdoors athlete, a mountain climber who intends to conquer the seven major summits of the world. I told her, "Look, Sandy, we're here for an hour; I can't possibly spend all this time on your hand. With it broken, you can't have been doing much the past few weeks; spring is coming and you're going to want to get outside."

She replied, "Radu, I'm not into this cosmetic nonsense."

"But you don't understand; the swimmer trains on the deck when the pool is frozen," I told her.

Still not quite believing that I would have her do anything more than lie on her side and work her abductors, Sandy agreed to let me train her more thoroughly. I had her running, jumping, and climbing the stall bars. I transformed my gym into an improvised outdoor scenario; imagining that she would have to step on unstable rocks during difficult hikes, I lined up medicine balls along the floor and made her walk on them. Sandy was fascinated by this athletic approach to training, and we became great friends; we hiked and climbed together, and she introduced me to what is now my greatest passion, kayaking.

With these exercises in hand you can imagine yourself training right there along with me and Matthew Broderick or Cindy Crawford. This may sound silly, but visualization is an important technique for all of my students. As you will soon read, it's this kind of imaging process that let Cindy Crawford outperform her own expectations while filming *Fair Game*. Mental representation leads to physical execution. So maybe one of these stories will help to imprint that you-can-do-it attitude in your heart and mind. Just like you, some of the most famous people in the world went to meet challenges in their lives a little unprepared, a little uneasy, or even a little shy. I want you to envision all of us there together, working hard, having fun, and doing what once seemed impossible.

But first I have to give you the same lecture that I give all my special students. Although personal training is a great way of focusing on body parts that need special attention or preparing for specific challenges, you'll benefit most from these specialized moves by incorporating them into a good overall conditioning program. I expect my personal training students to attend my Class just like all my other students, and I am going to expect the same of you. So please use these moves in conjunction with a regular exercise routine that includes either the Class or the Ultimate Challenge.

Success in training comes from breaking the pattern.

Cindy Crawford

When Cindy decided to play the part of a Miami district attorney in the 1995 thriller *Fair Game* with William Baldwin, we talked about how to prepare. I told her, "As a hero on the screen, you will have to look sexy, but you will have to perform." I knew I needed to talk to the stunt coordinator to find out exactly what Cindy would have to do in the film in order to figure out how she should train for it. I was more interested in what Cindy's character, a very athletic attorney, would do than in what Cindy the actress would do. But when I spoke to the stunt coordinator, he didn't understand; he said, "Just keep her strong and toned. Don't worry about it." I realized that we weren't going to have a team talk; that Cindy and I were going to have to plan it out.

After reading the script, she told me her character was going to have to perform a running escape, jump onto a moving train, and punch somebody out. To be credible, I believe actors should be able and willing to perform their own stunts, at least within reason. But many of the stunts in *Fair Game* were big risks, ones too big for Cindy to take. "Okay," I said, "I understand you don't have to perform, but we're going to change your routine to be very athletic." Even though Cindy wasn't going to do her own stunts, I wanted her to be capable of doing them, to know what it is like to hit someone hard, or to leap from the ground onto a moving train—and to look like someone capable of pulling off these moves.

I knew the director would have Cindy do the lead-up to each stunt; she would need to appear to be on the brink of doing something spectacular and breathtaking. But I also knew that actually trying

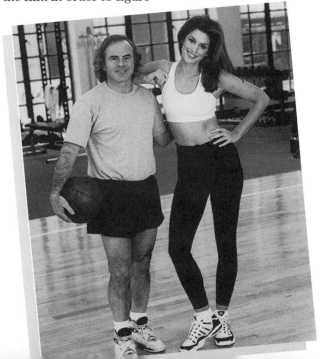

something is a lot different from just pretending; it adds a new dimension to how you think and how you carry yourself. You get the attitude of "I can do this," and it shows in your demeanor. We began training on the stall bars, the mats, the rings. I made her do pad work, punching and kicking pads that I held in my hands. I taught her to punch hard enough to bring a man down.

Cindy understood what I was doing with her training, but the tricky part came when she went off to shoot the movie. She had a trainer on location, who I knew would only focus on keeping her looking good, not on training her for performance. I didn't want the other trainer's aesthetics-based workouts to derail my teaching. So I told her to continue some of the things we did in the gym, like running, jumping, and skipping, on her own. By taking these elements of her training with her, she could remember our gym and the Radu way.

My little trick worked. One night I had a bad dream that Cindy had broken her leg, and I was so worried that I called her first thing in the morning and told her assistant about it. When she called me back she said, "Radu, it's amazing you had this dream! I'm okay, but you won't

believe this! Remember the stunt where my character jumps onto a train? When we were shooting, the director asked me to run alongside the train and stop at a certain point. But when I started running, I heard your voice in my head, urging me on, and I thought, 'I've done this with Radu, only it was much harder. I can do it here.' And I jumped onto that train!"

Cindy is a hard worker. If you give her something to do, and the guidance and instruction she needs to do it, she will hammer away at it until she gets it right—or better than right. She's a perfectionist who expects nothing but success of herself, and she is used to coming out on top. But when she leaped onto that train in front of the cast and crew of *Fair Game*, she surprised even herself. I had given her the tools to achieve, and she used those tools to accomplish more than was expected of her, and more than she expected of herself.

That is a beautiful thing about the process of getting fit, the way the benefits of your hard work suddenly spring up in your daily life. Of course you will get much satisfaction every time you're able to add another rep to your routine, or run an extra mile. But the big payoff comes when, just like Cindy, all of a sudden you can do

with ease things that you never thought you could do, or that were always a struggle before you began exercising. To give you an idea of how seriously Cindy trains three to four times per week, take a look at a sample of her Daily Log below.

CINDY'S DAILY LOG

9:00–9:30 Run outside or on the treadmill, or use the step machine for cardio training and to warm up.

9:30–10:00 Leg work: swings, lunges, running drills, skipping, hopping, broad jumps, squats, or special drills required for special projects.

10:00–10:30 Upper body: variations of push-ups and pull-ups, weight training using barbell and dumbbells, medicine ball, boxing/karate, calisthenics.

10:30–10:45 Waist: abdominal and lower-back exercises.

10:45–11:00 Stretching and a brief massage.

If a special project is in the works, we add obstacle courses, gymnastics, and kick boxing to our program. The time, intensity, volume, and complexity of the exercises is increased also.

Try the following exercises, which I include in Cindy's workout to give her power and strength in her thighs and buttocks (a sensitive area even for her, as it is for many women). For each exercise, do three sets of ten, fifteen, twenty, or twenty-five reps.

1.
Knee-to-chest swings

Stand arm's length from a wall, placing both hands on the wall for support. Bring your right knee toward your chest, then swing and extend straight behind you. Return to start and continue swinging the leg forward and back in a continuous movement. After completing one set, switch legs and repeat.

2.
Lateral leg swings

Stand arm's length from a wall and place both hands on the wall for support. Cross your right foot in front of your body, then swing it straight out to the side. Swing the leg from side to side in a continuous motion. Switch legs and repeat.

3.
Front-and-back swings

Stand with your left hand on a wall, chair, or tree for support, your right arm relaxed. Lift your right leg in front of your body, then swing it back behind you, keeping the knee slightly bent. Swing the leg forward and back in a continuous motion. Switch sides and repeat.

4.
Hurdles

Stand with both hands on the back of a chair, a full arm's length away. Lift your right leg with the knee bent; bring the leg forward, then extend it behind you and to the side. Switch legs and repeat.

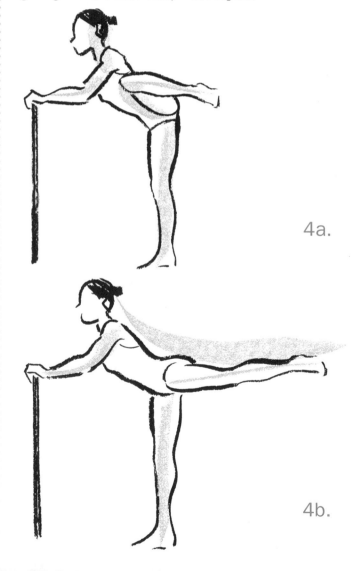

4a.

4b.

5.

Shot-put lunges

Begin by lunging to the right, right leg forward and knee bent, left leg extended behind you. Reach forward with your left arm and bend your right arm so that your right hand is next to your right ear. Spring up and reverse position, changing your weight to your left leg. With both legs straight, bring your right arm around to extend it in front of you, as if throwing a shot put. Spring up to return to start and repeat. Complete one set, switch sides and repeat.

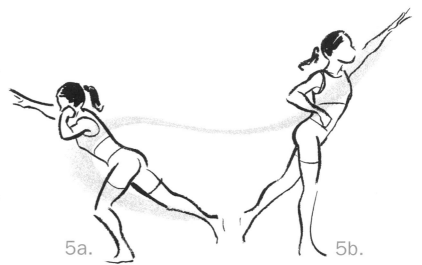

5a.
5b.

6.

Plié squats

Stand with legs wide, toes pointing out, arms resting on thighs. Squat down as far as you can, allowing your hands to slide to your knees; do not let your knees extend past your toes. As you return to standing, contract your buttocks and press down through your heels.

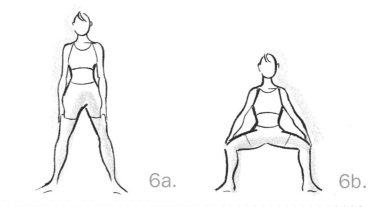

6a.
6b.

7.

Pelvic thrusts

Lie on your back, left knee bent, right ankle on left knee, arms by your sides. Keeping your abs tight and your pelvis tucked, lift your hips toward the ceiling, then return to starting position.

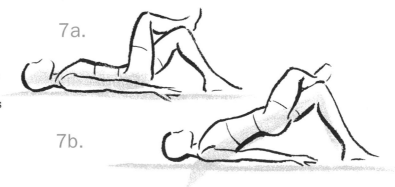

7a.
7b.

Regis
Philbin

Regis Philbin made a New Year's resolution to "get back the abs I had when I was seventeen." In typically outspoken fashion, he made this resolution on the air, on his morning talk show *Live with Regis and Kathie Lee*, and decided to broadcast his progress to his viewers. Regis's executive producer, Michael Gelman, was interviewing hot trainers in New York for the task, and he asked me to meet with Regis. During the interview, Regis mentioned that he had a back problem. I pointed out that I would have to tailor his program accordingly and said, "Regis, I can give you great abs, but I also have to get your back stronger and lessen its pain while doing that. After all, you are as weak as your weakest part." That got me the job.

Regis and I announced the challenge—to give Regis washboard abs—on the air with great fanfare. Behind the scenes, however, the job was frustrating. The producers just wanted me to come to the studio every day after the show and coach Regis for half an hour in his office. Their only goal was for Regis's abs to gain some definition, so that they would look ripply and "cut." On top of that, Regis is a very busy man, and there were constant distractions—phone messages, people wandering in to talk. I have to hand it to him, he kept on doing his crunches through it all.

Of course, you know by now that focusing on the cosmetic effects of exercise runs counter to everything I believe in. Naturally I didn't let on that I was impatient with the project; you have to play the part the way it's given to you. And at this point, Regis and I had not made the personal connection that is so crucial to good training.

After a couple of weeks I got my big break—at Regis's expense, but what happened was good for him in the long run. He threw out his back, and Michael asked me if I could help. I went straight to Regis's house and stretched and massaged him. While I was there, I said, "Regis, it's very difficult to work one part of your body. It's not going to fall into place this way. We're just addressing your waist, but there is so much more. You have to meet Radu, and you cannot meet Radu in this room or in your office."

"That means I have to come to the gym," he said.

"I'm afraid so," I replied.

Little did Regis know my gym would become his home away from home. He was there at least every other day. We kept up the abdominal work, but now the program became more serious, more well rounded. We got his abs looking great for the show, but now Regis had a more important personal goal at stake, and he kept working out after the public challenge was over.

I started to train him for tennis and other sports, and he turned into a real family member at the gym. One day Regis was shooting hoops with one of my instructors, Boris, a short, stocky Russian weight lifter who didn't know anything about basketball. Regis was having a great time with him: "Boris, you cannot shoot a basketball. You are a Russian box!" But Regis is kind and turned teacher to give Boris some pointers.

Inspired by his new regimen, Regis turned himself into a real expert and talked all the time on his show about what great shape he was in and how well his program was developing. My gym even became the setting for some episodes of his show. Regis and Cindy got to be great pals while working out together at my place, and one morning they exercised and chatted together on the air.

One day all this chatting almost got Regis into some trouble. An American Gladiator named Lace wrote to challenge him to a pull-ups contest. In typical competitive Regis style, he accepted—on the air. Only then did he realize what he'd done and came to the gym in a bit of a panic. "Radu, me and my big mouth. I get a letter from this female athlete, challenging me to pull-ups, and I accept in front of millions of people. How many do you think I can do?"

"Oh, about six," I told him. And Regis said, "That woman will eat me up. I hear she does sets of 12."

Kidding aside, I knew there had to be a way to get Regis through this mess. Problem solving is a lot of what physical training is all about—sizing up the strengths and weaknesses and making the best of what is there. Once I thought about it a little, I found the answer. "Reege," I said, "relax. Trust me. You're going to win this. We're going to do horizontal pull-ups."

My idea was to train him in a way that used the muscles differently from standard pull-ups, the kind that Lace would no doubt be practicing. For horizontals, you grip a bar above your chest and place your feet on a bench or chair so that your body is straight and parallel to the floor. You pull yourself up this way. It's a beautiful illustration of how specificity of training can give an athlete a competitive edge: you must train your muscles in the precise ways in which you're going to need them.

After Regis and I trained for a couple of weeks, Lace came on the show, dressed in her gladiator garb, totally confident. Backstage, I told her we would have to do horizontal pull-ups, because verticals were dangerous for Regis's back. Lace agreed; I'm sure she figured she could beat someone like Regis at just about any physical test.

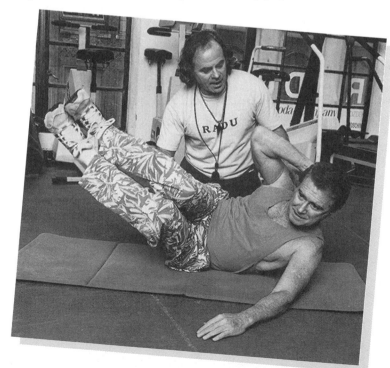

Then came the show-down: Lace went first. Gelman had rigged up a low trapeze bar on the set, but it was pretty high, so instead of propping them on a chair, I held Lace's feet so that her body was straight and parallel to the floor. Lace started the pull-ups. After three, I could feel her feet digging into my hands; I knew she was losing it already! She eked out about nine more, stopping around twelve or fourteen, exhausted.

Then it was Regis's turn. One pull-up, two. Kathie Lee was in heaven, figuring she was going to have something to hold over Regis for the next month. Three, four, five, six. He made it to the magic twelve and kept going! He was still flying after twenty-five pull-ups and nowhere near maxing out. The audience was loving it. Regis stopped and said to me and Kathie Lee, "Is this enough?" I could tell he had more in him. Physical training literally is touchy work: by using your hands on your students, you not only guide them through the correct and complete range of motion, but you also get feedback from their muscles. (You can do this for yourself to some extent: When you do abdominal work, for instance, place one hand on your abdomen; you'll be able to feel the muscles contract.) So I could tell that Regis was still going strong. I called out to the audience: "Do you need more? Who wants more?"

Sometimes I believe in my students more than they believe in themselves. Regis thought he would never be able to do more than a few pull-ups, but I wasn't about to let him get away with that kind of negative thinking. The only way you can fail is if you don't try or don't believe. If you don't try, and fail, I fail too. Personal training is all about teamwork: I give you all I've got, you give me all you've got, and we win. That's the way it is with Reege and me: everything he sets out to do, he accomplishes, and more.

In January of 1990, when he underwent surgery to correct a blocked artery in his heart, Regis knew that he would have to revamp his workout to include more aerobic exercise—which, incidently, he hated. After he recovered, he started power walking, using the time to come up with plans for future shows; the experience turned him into an exercise expert of sorts, and he put out a video inspired by his self-training and his workouts with me.

Regis can be an inspiration to all of us. He started on fitness again a little late in the game, but that was no obstacle. He'd been a great athlete at Notre Dame. I've included Regis's Daily Log to the left and some great ab work to the right.

REGIS'S DAILY LOG

1:30–2:00 Run or power walk on the treadmill for cardio training and to warm up.

2:00–2:30 Leg work: swings, lunges, squats, leg extensions and flexions, stretching.

2:30–3:00 Upper body: chest and shoulders one day, back and arms the next, alternating days.

3:00–3:15 Waist: abdominal and lower-back work.

3:15–3:30 If there's time, practice basketball shots; also stretching (although Regis doesn't have much patience with it).

Regis wanted great abs, and with the exercises that follow, he got them—as you will by incorporating this routine into your regular workout. He also turned his life around with the joy and rewards of a solid exercise program.

1.

Broomstick twists

Stand, feet slightly wider than shoulder-width apart, knees relaxed. Hold a broomstick behind your neck and twist from side to side, keeping your hips facing forward. Do six to ten reps.

2.

Elbow-to-knee lifts

Standing, place your hands behind your neck and bring your right elbow down toward your left knee while bringing the knee up toward the elbow. Return to start and repeat with left elbow and right knee. Continue alternating sides without stopping until you have done six to ten reps on each side.

3.

Side bends

Stand, feet wide, knees relaxed and slightly bent. Hold a dumbbell in each hand, arms at sides. Bend your torso to the left, bringing your right elbow toward the ceiling, then return to start. Continue bending from side to side until you have completed ten reps in each direction.

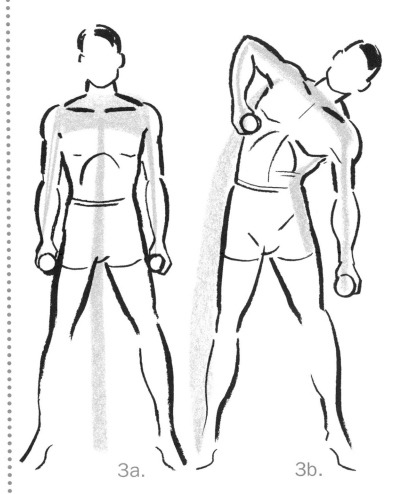

3a.

3b.

4.

Crunches

Lie on your back, knees bent, feet flat on floor. Place both hands behind your head, elbows out; press your lower back into the floor by tightening your abdominals and curling your pelvis toward the ceiling. Without allowing your back to lose contact with the floor, lift your head and shoulders about three inches, keeping your eyes focused on the ceiling and your elbows back. Lower your head and shoulders and repeat ten to twenty-five times. Then, maintaining the position of your back on the floor, do ten to twenty-five crunches to the right, leading each "lift" with your left shoulder. Switch sides and do ten to twenty-five crunches to the left; finish with another set of ten to twenty-five crunches to the center. Adding twists at the end will also strengthen your sides.

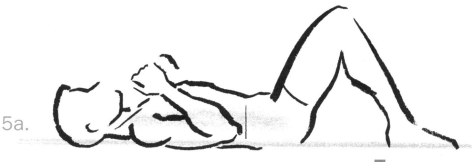

5a.

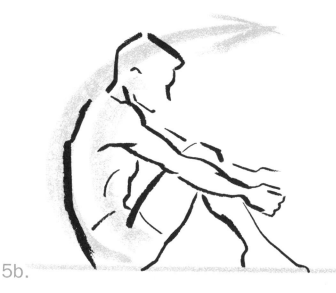

5b.

5.

Sit-ups

Lie on your back, knees bent, feet flat on the floor. Sit up slowly by bringing first your head, then your neck, and then each vertebra off the floor; imagine your torso as a piece of tape being peeled off the floor from one end. As you come to sitting position, bring both arms forward, stretching them past your shins. Reverse the move to return to start, lowering yourself one vertebra at a time and bringing your arms to your sides on the floor. Do ten to twenty-five reps.

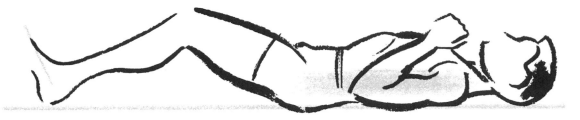

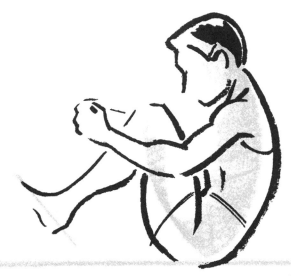

6a.

6b.

6.

Tuck jackknives

Lie on your back, arms bent at sides, hands fisted. Bend your legs slightly, feet together and heels on the floor. Sit up, letting arms extend forward as necessary and bringing both knees to your chest. Return to start slowly, holding your abdominals tight as you lower your torso and legs. Do ten to twenty-five reps.

7.

Lateral reaches

Lie on your back, arms out to the sides, legs together. Lift your left leg into the air while reaching toward it with your right hand, then return to start and repeat on the other side. Do ten to twenty-five reps on each side.

8.

Opposite arm and leg lift

Lie on your stomach with your legs straight and both arms extended overhead. Raise your left leg and right arm at the same time, then lower them. Do all reps on one side before switching to the other. Do ten to twenty-five reps on each side.

9.

Kneeling arm and leg lift

Kneel on hands and knees, neck aligned with spine (face the floor but do not drop your head down). Lift your right arm and extend it in front of you, while at the same time lifting your left leg and extending it behind you; hold this position for a count of three, lifting both arm and leg as high as you can without allowing your lower back to arch; tightening your abdominals will help. Return to kneeling and repeat with the other arm and leg. Do ten to twenty-five reps on each side.

10.

Arch

Lie facedown on floor, arms and legs extended. Carefully raise your head and both arms and both legs as high as possible and hold for a count of three. Lower and repeat, six to ten times.

11.

Cat stretch

Kneel on floor, head down and relaxed. Inhaling, tighten your abs and round your back toward the ceiling like an angry cat. Exhale and return to starting position. Do ten to twenty-five reps.

12.

Sideways over-thigh stretch

Kneel on floor and stretch back over your thighs, arms on the floor in front of you and to the side. Shift your weight to the right side and then to the left, holding stretch for 10 seconds.

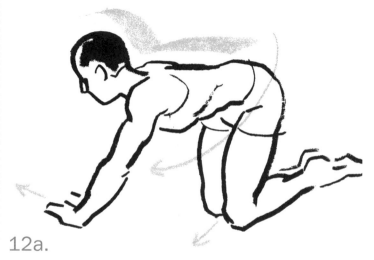

12a.

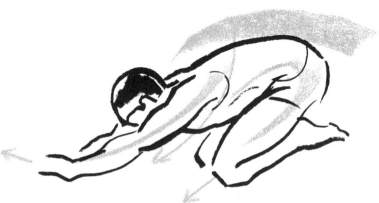

12b.

Regis's Triceps Definers

Regis loves to have a lot of definition and bulk in his triceps. It's a part of his body he really enjoys training. These are three of his favorite moves. Do three sets of four reps if you're just beginning, three sets of six reps if you've been working out for a while, and three sets of eight to ten reps if you're an advanced exerciser, using the heaviest weight you can handle for each move.

1. BEHIND-THE-NECK TRICEPS EXTENSIONS: Hold a dumbbell in your right hand at the top, so that the wider part of the weight is resting in your hand. Hold the dumbbell behind your head with your elbow pointing straight up. This is a harder version of the classic behind-neck extension, in which you would use your left hand to steady your right arm: I want that right arm to do the work of maintaining the position, so place your left hand on your waist or relax it by your side. Straighten, and then lower, your right arm without allowing the upper arm to move.

2. KICK BACKS: Holding a dumbbell in your right hand, bend at the hips to rest your left forearm on your bent left knee; extend your right leg behind you. Bend your right arm so that the elbow points toward the ceiling. Without moving your upper arm, exhale and straighten your right elbow to bring the weight behind you. Inhale as you return to starting position.

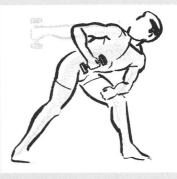

3. HEAD CRUSHERS: Lie on your back, knees bent, feet together. Grasp the ends of one dumbbell in each hand and position it above your forehead, elbows pointing toward the ceiling. Keeping your upper arms steady, straighten your elbows, then return to start.

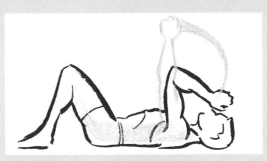

Matthew Broderick

Matthew Broderick came to me with a nutty goal: he needed to lose some weight for a movie, but the part also called for him to look like a weakling. I said, "Hey, I can't do that. You don't come to me to make yourself look sick! Leave that up to the makeup person." Instead we set out to get Matthew into better shape, increase his endurance, tone up his muscles—general physical conditioning.

The secret of good training depends on two things: knowing your goals, as I've already discussed, and figuring out what it takes to motivate yourself to get there. It's different for everyone. Cindy trusted me, her friend, to know what work was needed for her movie role, and she wanted to get it right. Regis had the pressure of millions of viewers watching, but his health became the ultimate inducement to exercise when both his back and his heart gave him trouble. His goals became much

more critical, and the results much more significant.

Matthew was a tougher proposition, because he's a shy, modest guy, a very private person. If someone else came into the gym, I could tell Matthew would feel self-conscious and not work as hard. He was not completely confident about his physical abilities. It is important for a trainer to develop a real rapport with a student, to gain that person's trust. Matthew and I did a lot of talking, as I tried to find experiences we both shared and could relate to. That was the first step. We had to become friends.

The next task was to figure out how to motivate Matthew to work his hardest, and what might stand in the way of his achievement. It's a little bit like being a doctor, and every student needs a different prescription. Matthew needed a cure for his discomfort in the gym, so that he could block everything else out and concentrate on his program. I

came up with a bold way of curing this.

On a day when there were a lot of women in the gym, exactly the kind of crowd that would make Matthew hold back because he knew those women would be watching him, I got him to try something new and sort of strange. I tossed him a medicine ball and had him lie down on his back in front of the basketball goal. From there he had to do a sit-up and, as soon as he was all the way up, shoot the medicine ball into the hoop over his head. I made him show off!

I use the trick of mixing familiar moves all the time. It's a great way to prepare the body for the unexpected; that's what life's all about, after all. If you merely make a body strong and beautiful, without making it work better in the real world, then what have you got? A perfect little doll you pick up and say, "Isn't that pretty?" and then put down. There's no other use for it. In fact, that's how Cindy Crawford is different from so many other models. They all look the part, but they don't have the athletic attitude Cindy has. And because she has that, she carries herself with confidence; she's ready for whatever life throws her.

Matthew needed that kind of confidence, and the best way to get it was to shock it out of him. He got caught up in the challenge of throwing that medicine ball through the hoop, which is hard work. The man had to do a sit-up holding an eight-pound ball, then throw it high into the air, which required great upper-body strength. Not only that, he had to call on his hand-eye coordination to get the ball into the basket. He made eight out of ten shots like this, and jumped up smiling. It was an epiphany for him to do something physically difficult in front of a lot of people.

After that, Matthew stopped doubting himself, and his self-confidence grew along with his strength and endurance.

I found that if I ever thought he was holding back, I could tease him into performing. "Hey, Matthew, out late last night, huh? Well, you play last night, you pay today!" He'd then work twice as hard to prove me wrong. He had that much confidence and pride about what he could do; he went from being self-conscious about his physical capabilities to being competitive about them.

Here's Matthew's Daily Log, to give you an idea of how he developed. Physically, Matthew grew in many ways. His arms became really strong, and the most amazing transformation took place in his legs. He was already a bike rider, but after training, he got so strong that he literally outgrew the bike he owned; it just didn't challenge him anymore. So he bought a beautiful all-terrain bike that lets him go all over the place—up steep hills and into rocky areas where you need a lot of power to push through. Just as he conquered the realm of his own self-doubt, he is conquering the physical world.

MATTHEW'S DAILY LOG

11:00–11:40 After a few minutes of general warm-up, we would do Radu-Running (for details, see pages 123–124), plus skips, hops, broad jumps, kangaroo jumps, deep jumps from a bench, into a broad jump, into a high jump over an obstacle or another bench. And more lunges, squats, and benchwork.

11:40–11:45 Waist: broomstick twists, crunches, and reverse leg curls.

11:45–12:00 Arms: pull-ups and push-ups.

12:00–12:20 Chest and shoulders or back and arms, using the barbell, dumbbells, pulleys, and elastics on alternating days.

12:20–12:30 Waist and more abdominal work.

12:30–12:45 Medicine ball, basketball shots, stretching.

These are the exercises that give Matthew's lower body the strength he needs to power that bike off the beaten path, and maybe they can do the same for you as well. Have fun showing off!

1.
Half-squats down
Stand, feet shoulder-width apart, toes forward, arms at sides. Squat halfway down, bringing your arms out in front of you, then return to standing. Squat up and halfway down six times. On the last rep, go to a full squat and immediately begin the following half-squats up.

2.
Half-squats up
From full squat position, come halfway up, then squat back down; repeat six times. Follow half-squats up with six reps of full squats, going through the full range of motion—or complete six reps of legs together squats.

3.
Legs together squats
Squat, feet together and both hands on floor a few inches in front of toes. Straighten both legs, keeping your hands on the floor (or as close as possible.) Squat up and down in a controlled, unbroken movement six times.

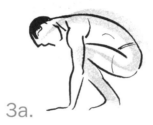

3a.

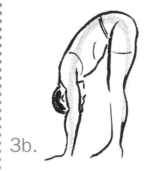

3b.

4.
Giant steps
In an area where you have room to "travel," take six giant steps forward by bringing your right knee high, extending your leg, and stepping far forward into a lunge, then repeating the move with your left leg.

5.
Broad jumps with two leaps
Stand, legs together, arms at your sides. Bend your knees deeply, bring both arms behind you, and jump forward as far as you can, swinging your arms forward for momentum. Take two smaller jumps backward. Repeat the sequence six times.

6.
Basketball jumps
Stand, hands in front of chest as if holding a basketball. Bend your knees and spring up as high as you can, lifting both arms into the air as if shooting the ball. Land softly, allowing your knees to bend again, and jump back up. Repeat ten, fifteen, or twenty times.

Matthew's Biceps Curls

In addition to his lower body work, Matthew trains his upper body rigorously with the three exercises below and others. If you do these three variations on the biceps curl, you'll soon develop terrific, solid, graceful-looking upper arms. The curls will strengthen as well as define your biceps. Do three sets of four reps if you're just beginning; three sets of six if you consider yourself intermediate; three sets of eight to ten if you're strong. Choose the heaviest weight you can handle to complete a full set of reps at whatever your level.

1. ALTERNATING CURLS: Stand with feet comfortably apart, knees relaxed. Hold a dumbbell in each hand in front of your thighs, palms facing forward. Bend your left arm to bring the dumbbell to your shoulder, contracting your biceps as you lift, then slowly straighten your left arm while bending your right one. Continue alternating right and left without stopping.

2. PREACHER CURLS: Sit on a chair, your left arm resting on your left knee, your left hand on your right thigh. Holding a weight, extend your right arm toward the floor in front of you, resting it against your left hand for support. Your palm should be facing out. Bring the weight to your shoulder, then slowly lower it, resisting the pull of gravity on the return.

3. SQUAT CURLS: Assume a half-squat, feet wide, holding a dumbbell in each hand

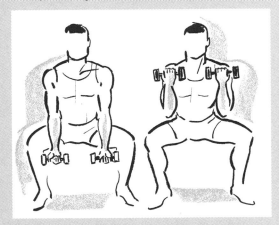

between your legs, arms straight and palms facing forward and hanging free. Do one set of curls in this position, then return to standing for a brief rest between sets. Better yet, try alternating curls; if you do choose to alternate, time your breathing to either arm's curls.

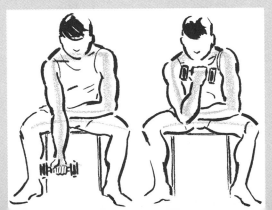

Vanessa Williams

When I take on the challenge of training an actor for a part, I have to know exactly what the part will be. With Cindy's character in *Fair Game*, I had to do some second-guessing, but when Vanessa Williams sought my help for her role as the lead in the Broadway hit *Kiss of the Spider Woman*, my work was cut out for me. The role required her to be able to jump and leap and climb, and to do so with the grace and ease of a spider.

Not only that, but this had to be Vanessa's spider. She was following in the footsteps of Chita Rivera, who originated the role, and Vanessa needed to make the character her own. When I began to create Vanessa's spider in my mind, I started thinking in terms of another animal—the cat. Cats are natural gymnasts; they are acrobats. They have the sense of balance and the agility and grace to ignore every rule of gravity, and like Vanessa, they are very sensual. So I envisioned her spider as catlike, a tigress or a panther, with the same sort of unselfconscious agility. I never discussed this vision with Vanessa. It would have intellectualized the process too much and made her self-conscious; I wanted her to feel, not think. (Matthew Broderick might have balked at shooting hoops with a medicine ball if I had given him time to think.) I wanted to go straight to Vanessa's muscles and give them a feel for moving like a cat.

I asked her to move in unexpected ways, backward, through the air, sideways. I had her crawl on the floor. Each time she surprised her body by taking it in new directions. I had her do simple gymnastics moves, like cartwheels and handstands, to bring back some of the feelings she had doing these tricks as a child. I also wanted her to experience the sensation of moving through the air, as a cat does when it leaps impossibly long distances, or a spider does as it is suspended in the air while spinning its web. There wasn't time to teach Vanessa to do aerial flips and handsprings, so I did the next best thing. In the course of our training, I would simply flip her over, forward or backward, in the air. She wasn't doing it on her own, but she felt what it was like.

In three months, she had become that beautiful spider, in her heart and mind as well as physically. It showed in her eyes and in the remarkable poise with which she carried herself.

Here are some of the moves that turned Vanessa into an agile, graceful spider, and which you can use in your own training to enhance your balance and coordination. Be free with these moves, incorporating them into your running routine, or doing them whenever you're outside with plenty of space and a level surface to move on.

Do the following exercises in whatever order you'd like, but try to maintain each for ten or fifteen seconds before changing direction. Do three sets of each.

1.
Sashays
Move sideways by lunging to the right with your right leg, arms relaxed. Bring your left foot toward the right one; as they meet, leap up a few inches, reaching both arms up. Repeat this move immediately upon landing; continue sashaying to the right in a flowing, unbroken movement before switching directions.

2.
Sideways running
Run sideways, bringing your knees up high.

3.
Backward running
Pick an area where you feel safe moving backwards with a minimum of head turning, and run, elbows bent at your sides.

4.
Stag leaps
Run, then leap, extending your legs straight in front of and behind you.

5.
Criss crosses
Run sideways to the right, leading with your right foot and crossing your left foot alternately in front and in back of the right one, then switch directions.

6.
Belly crawls
Lie on your belly on the floor, arms extended in front of you. Wriggle forward by reaching forward with your right arm and then your left, rocking your torso from side to side for momentum and bending your knees to bring your legs toward your elbows. Vanessa also crawled on her hands and feet, and you may wish to add that to your routine.

4.

John Kennedy Jr.

My first job as a trainer was as an assistant at the gym of Nicholas Kounovsky, an elite Russian fitness coach who specialized in Swedish gymnastics (as I would go on to do), believing that the grace of movement was more important than brute strength. If Jack LaLanne, a contemporary of Kounovsky's, was the J. C. Penney of fitness, then Kounovsky was the Neiman Marcus, and he attracted such students as Jacqueline Kennedy.

Eventually, Alex and Walter, two trainers under Kounovsky, opened their own gym, and brought me with them. It was a life-changing experience for me: I was a hotshot gymnastics instructor at Alex and Walter; I met my wife, Vicki, there, and developed a strong following of students. It was from that base that I left to open my own gym. By this time, a new generation of Kennedys was on the scene, embracing that love of sports for which the fam-

ily is famous in a contemporary way. And this younger crop of Kennedys—Lee Radziwill, her son Anthony, Caroline, and, of course, John—all found their way to the next generation of fitness training at my gym.

Like all the Kennedys, John has always been very athletic. He loves kayaking, swimming, biking, and touch football, and although he looks great, when he comes to me the emphasis of his training is very much on performance. John's a great example of someone who is disciplined to keep himself in a constant state of physical readiness. He is one of those students who actually follows my advice and takes regular classes to maintain a solid foundation of overall fitness. I encourage you to do the same with your program. This way John has a solid base to build on when a special challenge comes his way; for him, that's usually a sports expedition—a biking trip or a kayaking excursion.

In fact, the times I'm

most likely to interact with John is when he has an adventure to go on. He'll come in and say, "Hey, Radu, I'm going kayaking in the Red Sea. Gotta get in shape." Then I tell him what he needs to do, and he has the knowledge—of exercise and his own body's power and limitations—to go off on his own and do it. He's always functioning at 80 percent of his physical potential, so that when a new and exciting challenge or task comes his way, it is nothing for him to bring himself to 100 percent to meet that challenge. By contrast, I train a boxer who was recently in a panic because he was facing a big match and knew he wasn't prepared. He would call me to complain: "I don't have the endurance. I can't do it." All I could say to him was "Why didn't you do what I said, man, and run?" The boxer didn't remain anywhere near 80 percent of his capacity, so it was too hard for him to build back up to 100 percent in time for his match. I'm sorry to say that he paid the price and lost his first bout ever featured on HBO.

John Kennedy doesn't want to let a great opportunity—which for him is a chance to play and explore outdoors—pass him by, so he stays ready at all times. His upper body is what gives him his signature physique—but it's also what allows him to function as an athlete. The following are among his favorite moves, which, combined, give his upper body volume and bulk, as well as muscle strength and endurance. Even if you can't live John's lifestyle, you can still sport the same strength and healthy look.

Here are some of the weight exercises John does to prepare for kayaking trips and to maintain his general health. Aside from dumbbells, you will need access to a barbell and a lat-pulldown machine. Do three sets of four reps if you're beginning; three sets of six if you consider yourself intermediate; three sets of eight to ten if you're strong. Choose the heaviest weight you can handle to complete a full set of reps; the last two should take you to exhaustion.

1.

Bench press

Lie on your back on a bench, knees bent, feet flat. Tighten your abs and press your lower back into the bench. Ask a spotter to hand you the barbell nested above your chest; hold it about an inch above your collarbone, hands slightly wider than your shoulders. Exhale and straighten both arms toward the ceiling, keeping the bar even and being careful to not let your wrists bend backward. Inhaling, slowly lower the bar to your chest.

2.

Lateral flyes

With bent knees, lie on your back, a dumbbell in each hand and positioned over your chest. Face palms inward and bend elbows slightly so they point to the

sides. Press your lower back into the bench. Inhaling, open your arms and lower the weights to the sides without altering the bent-elbow position of your arms, until you feel a stretch across the front of your shoulders. Exhale and return the weights to start, contracting your chest as you lift.

3.

Pullovers

Lie on your back. Hold a dumbbell in each hand, knuckles facing in and close together, elbows slightly bent. Inhaling, bring both arms over your head as far as you can, tapping the weights lightly on the floor, then exhale and bring them back to starting position.

4.

Pull-downs

Sit up straight on a lat-pull-down machine, holding the bar with an overhand grip, hands wider than shoulders. Lean forward slightly, head in line with spine. Inhaling, pull the bar down as far as possible, squeezing your shoulder blades together. Exhale as you slowly allow your arms to straighten, controlling the bar until your arms are straight.

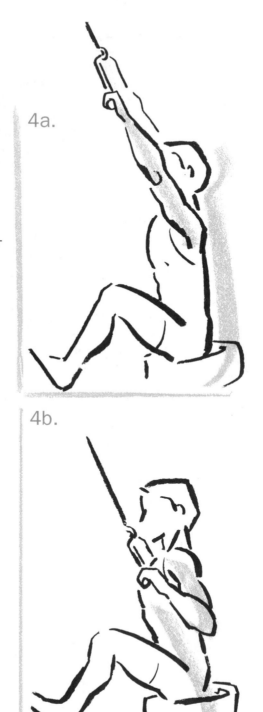

4a.

4b.

5.

Rowing

Kneel with your left knee and leg on a bench, your right foot flat on the floor. Holding a dumbbell in your right hand, tighten your abdominals and straighten your arm toward the floor. Exhaling, bend your elbow straight up toward the ceiling, bringing the dumbbell toward your armpit. Inhale and slowly straighten your arm.

6.

Overhead presses

Stand, a dumbbell in each hand, elbows bent and close to sides, the weights at shoulder level, palms facing forward. Press both weights toward the ceiling, exhaling and controlling the movement so that the weights stay even. Inhale and lower the weights to shoulder height.

7.

Sun fists

Stand, feet shoulder-width apart, knees relaxed, abdominals tight. Hold a dumbbell in each hand at chest level, palms facing in. Alternate punching your right and left hands straight in front of you without locking your elbows.

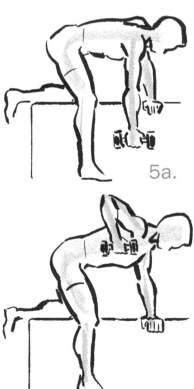

5a.

5b.

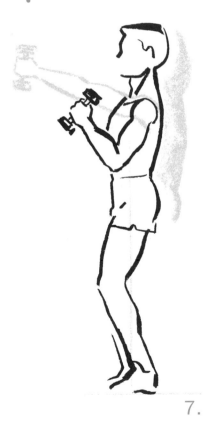

7.

Matthew
Modine

When actor Matthew Modine came in to train for *Cutthroat Island*, a big-budget pirate movie, he said, "Man, I've gotta take my top off and I've gotta look good." Period. That was it. Matthew is more of an actor than an action hero, and so he really needed to look the part. Leave the rest up to the stunt guy. So I designed a program to pump up the volume of his chest and arms. But that little voice inside me that's always pushing people for more kept saying, "Why am I wasting my time with this guy if all he wants is to beef up?"

It turns out we were on the same page, because as Matthew got stronger he began to think he could perform many of his own stunts. He knew his fight scenes would play much more credibly, and the camera could come in much tighter, if he were doing the work himself.

Just as I had created in my mind the sensual spider that Vanessa Williams was to become, I had to invent a pirate for Matthew. He told me his character would be climbing ladders, swinging from ropes, and engaged in swordplay. For Matthew to pull this off, we had to jazz up his routine quite a bit. I cut back on the heavy load work that we had been doing to bulk him up and put him on an extensive sequence of push-ups, pull-ups, and walking on his hands, plus some work on the gymnastics rings and ropes in my gym. A great Russian fencing coach named Yory came in to prepare him for the sword fights.

The fencing was great fun. At one point, a Hungarian fencer from my gym, the Russian coach, and I challenged Matthew to a duel. He was fighting off a Russian, a Romanian, and a Hungarian simultaneously! By the end of his training, Matthew Modine was not just a great-looking "posing" actor—he was a great-looking *functional* actor. And he felt, prepared for anything his role might demand.

MATTHEW'S DAILY LOG

10:00–10:30 Warm-up, Radu-Running (for more, see pages 123–124), drills, calisthenics, a few push-ups and pull-ups, some abdominal work for five minutes and lightweight medicine-ball work.

10:30–11:15 Fencing, sparring, fighting techniques, and multiple attacks.

11:15–11:30 Discussion and rest.

11:30–12:30 Legs: Skipping, hopping, broad jumps (similar to Matthew Broderick's routine), plus abdominal work for five minutes; then high-bar and floor gymnastics, ring work, climbing on one and then two ropes, rope ladder climbing techniques.

We finished with upper-body work (weights: chest and shoulders or back and arms on alternating days), more abdominal work for three to five minutes, medicine ball and basketball work, and stretching.

Matthew's real moment of triumph (and vicariously, mine) came during shooting, when he performed a stunt in which he caught his costar, Geena Davis, with one arm while balancing on a rope ladder. It took some amazing strength for him to pull it off—particularly since he had to do it, take after take. But Matthew told me that every time he caught Geena, he quietly whispered, "Thank you, Radu!"

Matthew's Daily Log will give an idea of how hard he worked—and how it can pay off for you, too.

You probably don't have to catch women one-handed as they fall through the air, and the demand for pirates is pretty slim these days, but it's great to have that kind of muscle strength and agility. This push-up/pull-up series will give you exactly that. Do three sets of four, six, or eight to ten reps, depending on your fitness level.

1.
Standard push-ups
Place your hands on the floor about shoulder-width apart, fingers pointing forward. Extend your legs behind you, feet together and balanced on toes. Make sure your head is in line with your spine. Tighten your abs and tuck your pelvis so that your body is straight from head to heels. Maintaining this position (don't release the tension in your abdominals so that your belly drops and your lower back collapses), bend your elbows until your chest is just a few inches from the floor, then push up through your arms to return to starting position.

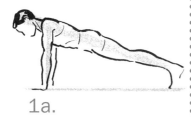

1a.

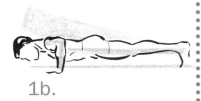

1b.

2.
Wide-arm push-ups
Assume the position described above, this time separating your hands a bit farther than shoulder-width apart, the fingers pointing out on a diagonal.

3.
Hands-together push-ups
Assume the standard push-ups position, hands right under your chest, fingers pointing in and touching, elbows out to the sides.

4.
See-saws
Assume position for standard push-ups. Lower your chest to the ground, but use only your right arm to lift your body up, then lower it back to the start. Next push up with your left arm. Continue shifting from side to side until you have completed all the reps on each arm.

5.

One-handed push-ups

Assume standard push-ups position, balancing on your right arm with your left hand behind your back. Do all reps with your right arm, then switch sides.

6.

Incline push-ups

Position your arms as for regular push-ups, your legs extended straight behind you and your feet resting on the seat of a chair. Lower your body to the floor and then return to start.

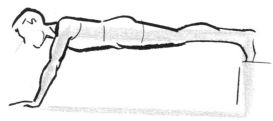

6a.

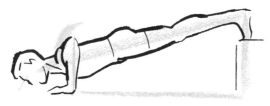

6b.

7.

Push-ups with a clap

Perform a regular push-up to the point at which your chest is near the ground. Push up hard enough to lift your body high enough into the air that you can bring your palms together for a loud clap, before you land in starting position, chest near the ground.

8.

Overhand pull-ups

Reach up and grasp a pull-ups bar with both hands, arms slightly wider than shoulders, fingers pointing forward. Cross your feet at the ankles if you wish, tighten your abs, and pull your body up so that the bar is just below your chin, then slowly straighten your arms.

9.

Underhand pull-ups

Grasp the pull-ups bar with your fingers pointing behind you and repeat move as described above.

10.

Over-under pull-ups

With your right hand, grasp the bar overhanded; with your left, hold on under-handed. Do one full set of reps in this position, then switch the direction of the hands for another full set of reps.

2.

Hip flexions

Stand, hands on hips, left leg straight, right leg slightly forward. Keeping your upper body straight, raise your right leg straight in front of you as high as you can. Lower the leg slowly, in a controlled motion. Switch sides and repeat.

3.

Knee extensions

Stand, right hand on a wall for support, left hand on hip. Lift your left knee to waist level. Without moving your left thigh, straighten the leg. As you bend and straighten the leg, keep your thigh as still as possible. Switch sides and repeat.

4.

Knee flexions

Stand straight with your right hand on a wall for support, your left hand on your hip. Bend left knee toward your buttocks; your calf should come to the back of your thigh at the top of the move. Lower and repeat, then switch sides.

5.

Abductors

Lie on your right side, head resting on right hand, left hand on floor in front of you for support. "Stack" your left leg directly on top of your right, pull in your abs and tuck your pelvis. Raise your left leg as high as you can, toes forward; do not lean back. Lower leg and repeat, then switch sides.

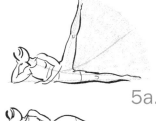

5a.

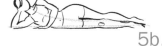

5b.

6.

Adductors

Lie on your right side, head resting on right hand, left hand on floor in front of you for support. Bend your left leg and place your left foot flat on the floor behind your right thigh. Raise your right leg straight up toward the ceiling, foot pointing forward. Lower and repeat, then switch sides

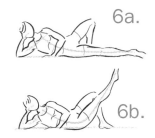

6a.

6b.

The Ultimate Challenge

Now it's time to get serious—I wasn't voted the Toughest Trainer in New York City for nothing. The Class served as the first step to total conditioning, but it is here that you will really test yourself.

Like the gymnastics coach whose ultimate goal is to teach a budding gymnast how to do a double-somersault with a twist, I start out with the basics. Just as he breaks the move down into its smallest elements, I provide no-frills exercise programs. It is only when the gymnast has perfected all these simple elements that he or she will be able to integrate them into a flawless double-somersault with a twist. It's like teaching Matthew Broderick a set of separate skills—to handle a medicine ball, shoot a basketball dead-on through the hoop, and execute a perfect sit-up—then *bam!* one day making him put it all together in a surprising and challenging new way. You

thought I simply wanted him to show off? No way. Matthew worked hard to do that exercise, and his body got as much exercise as his ego. You are ready for the Ultimate Challenge because you've either mastered the Class or opened this book already prepared and looking for a tougher challenge.

As I always say, people often don't have a clue of their ultimate potential until they try, and each success engenders a new goal. The physical potential of a healthy human body is amazing, almost infinite. As long as you continue to challenge it, it will continue to grow and change. That's why this is the workout for you: it's a master class for those of you who have exhausted the challenges of the Class and are ready to move on to the next level. These exercises are still based on moves you do every day, but they are more complex. Rather than simply squat, I will ask you to finish with a jump into the air. The chest presses now incorporate a twist of the forearms. The lateral raises will be executed behind your hips.

You see, I am melding and altering the simple skills you have mastered already, just as the gymnastics coach puts together the simple elements of a complex aerial somersault. Changing your routine is key to soaring to new heights of fitness and accomplishment. It is vital to preventing boredom. It is essential to keeping your mind open. The students who take my six o'clock master class have learned to expect the unexpected, because I'm not going to repeat the same routine from class to class.

This is the kind of routine that separates Radu from the rest. You won't get a workout like this anywhere else; it's the type of training my reputation is built upon. This is what it takes to soar to new heights of fitness and accomplishment, to become a Cindy Crawford or Matthew Modine and not just another pretty body. As you attempt this new program, a feeling of déjà vu may wash over you as you struggle to finish the minimum amount of reps for an exercise. It may remind you of how you felt when you tried the Class for the first time. Then, the strength of your dreams and desires kept you going; now, you are equipped with something more solid than a vision. You have lived the reality of success. You know you can do anything you put your mind to, including this class. Do it. Never be content. Celebrate where you are, but don't forget there's an even better you just over the horizon. I hope to meet you there again someday, where we can take on even greater challenges together, as coach and student— and as friends.

Each success engenders a new goal.

The Challenge
WARM UP

NECK
Consult a doctor if you experience prolonged dizziness.

1.
Stand with feet shoulder-width apart. Look up and down.
Reps: 6–10 each way
Sets: 1
Weights: None

2.
Look over each shoulder side to side.
Reps: 6–10 each way
Sets: 1
Weights: None

3.
Bring your ear to your left shoulder, then to your right.
Reps: 6–10 each way
Sets: 1
Weights: None

SHOULDERS
4.
Scissors
Swing left arm by your ear and right arm by your side, alternating arms continuously.
Reps: 6–10 each way
Sets: 1
Weights: None

5.
Crossovers
Cross your arms in front of your chest and swing them back out to sides, arms slightly bent and parallel to the floor.
Reps: 6–10 each way
Sets: 1
Weights: None

6.
Double arm rotations
Extend both arms out to the side, elbows slightly bent, in a relaxed position. Circle both arms forward; then circle them back.
Reps: 6–10 each way
Sets: 1
Weights: None

WAIST

7.

Side bends

Widen your stance slightly and bend at the waist to the right, keeping your lower body stable and bringing your left arm overhead. Switch directions and continue alternating right and left. Do not hold position; move continuously.

Reps: 6–10 each way
Sets: 1
Weights: None

8.

Waist twists

Cross arms in front of chest and grasp hands, keeping arms parallel to ground; twist right and left at waist continuously.

Reps: 6–10 each way
Sets: 1
Weights: None

9.

Back extensions

Standing with feet shoulder-width apart and knees slightly bent, bend your torso toward your toes, allowing your arms to relax down toward the floor. Stand up tall, reaching your arms toward the ceiling, then bend forward and down again in a continuous movement.

Reps: 4–10
Sets: 1
Weights: None

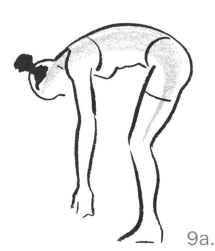

9a.

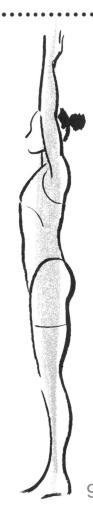

9b.

10.
Torso circles
Stand with feet shoulder-width apart, toes forward, knees relaxed. Place hands on hips, bend forward slightly at the waist, then move torso right, back, and left, making a full circle. Repeat all reps before changing direction.
Reps: 6–10 each way
Sets: 1
Weights: None

11.
Windmills
Stand, bending at waist, and touch right foot with left hand, then left foot with right hand, constantly swinging your arms to each foot. Your head and shoulders should follow the movement of the upper arm in order to increase range of motion.
Reps: 6–10 each way
Sets: 1
Weights: None

HIPS/KNEES
12.
Partial side lunges
Stand with feet slightly wider than shoulder-width apart, toes pointing forward, hands on knees. Keep your hip area tight and your shoulders relaxed. Bend your right leg and straighten your left, allowing the toes of your left foot to come off the floor; make sure that your right knee does not extend past your toes. Repeat on the other side, and continue alternating from right to left.
Reps: 6–10 each way
Sets: 1
Weights: None

13.
Deep side lunges
Widen stance and bend knees for deep side lunges to stretch inner thigh. Remain in deep lunge position and pulse slightly on each leg, then move on to lunge twists.
Reps: 6–10 each way
Sets: 1
Weights: None

14.
Lunge twists
Stand with your right knee bent, your left leg extended straight behind you, toes on floor. Place your hands on your hips. Jump lightly and turn in the air so that you land with your left knee bent and your right leg extended behind you. Continue jumping and twisting without pausing. After completing all reps of lunge twists, bring feet closer together and twist hips, hopping continuously.
Reps: 12–20 each way
Sets: 1
Weights: None

15.
Front lunges
Step forward with your left leg, keeping the knee bent slightly without stretching all the way to the floor; do not allow your left knee to extend past your toes. Let your right leg straighten naturally, with as wide a stance as possible for stretching hamstrings. Switch.
Reps: 6–10 each way
Sets: 1
Weights: None

EXERCISES

RUNNING

For confined area. If you have the space, run lightly around in circles or on a path. Repeat entire sequence twice, 20–30 seconds for each running exercise, and rest 60–90 seconds after each sequence.

16.

a. Run in place.
b. Run in place, knees up.
c. Run in place.
d. Run in place, heels to butt.
e. Run in place.
f. Jump up and down on both feet, arms reaching upward as if shooting a basketball.
g. Run in place.
h. Run in place with legs straight forward.
i. Run in place.
j. Run in place with legs straight back.
k. Run in place.
l. Jump in place and scissor legs forward quickly.
m. Run in place.
n. Run in place with legs straight, side to side.
o. Run in place.
p. Power skip, sharply and rhythmically.
q. Run in place.
r. Jump and twist your torso as you jump.
Reps: repeat entire sequence
Sets: 2
Weights: None

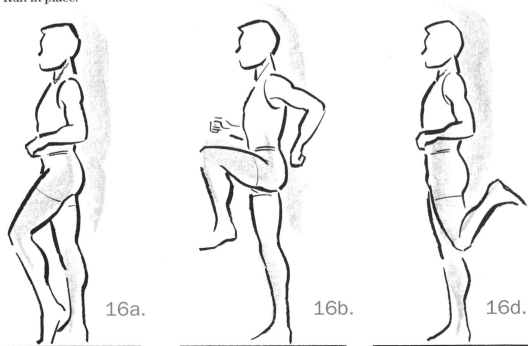

16a.   16b.   16d.

LEGS

17.

Front lunges

Stand, arms bent at waist level and shoulders relaxed. Lift your left leg, knee bent 90 degrees and thigh parallel to floor. Step far forward with your left leg, extending it and lowering your body toward the floor. Do not allow your left knee to extend past your toes. Your left heel should contact floor first, then rest of foot to toe in a rolling motion. Let your right leg straighten naturally, but firmly. Push back and up from your left toe to your heel, bringing your knee up to return to starting position. Complete 1 set on left leg, 1 set on right leg, then rest 10 to 15 seconds before beginning next set, starting with left leg again.

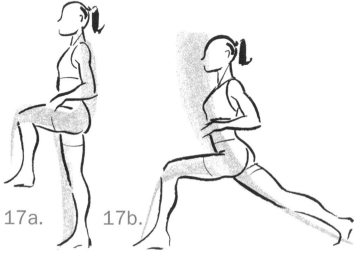

17a.   17b.

Reps: beginning 8
intermediate 10
advanced 12
Sets: 3
Weights: None

18.

Reverse lunges

Step back, extending left leg behind you. Lower your body toward the floor and reach your left leg as far back as it can go, then push up to starting position. The right knee should not extend past your toes. Complete 1 set on left leg, 1 set on right, then rest 10 to 15 seconds before starting with left leg again.

Reps: beginning 8
intermediate 10
advanced 12
Sets: 3
Weights: None

19.

Combination lunges

Combine both front and reverse lunge techniques by lunging forward then back with the same leg. As you return to starting position, bring your knee up and pause for a fraction of a second before going into next lunge. Complete 1 set with left leg, 1 set with right, then rest 10 to 15 seconds, before beginning next set on left leg. At end of all sets, rest 15 to 30 seconds by shaking legs out.

Reps: beginning 8
intermediate 10
advanced 12
Sets: 3
Weights: None

20.

Legs together squats

Squat, feet together and both hands on floor a few inches in front of toes. Straighten both legs, keeping your hands on the floor (or as close as possible). Squat up and down in a controlled, unbroken movement. Rest 15 to 20 seconds by shaking legs out.

Reps: beginning 8
intermediate 10
advanced 12

Sets: 1

Weights: None

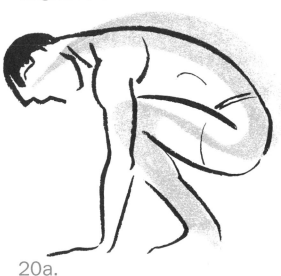

20a.

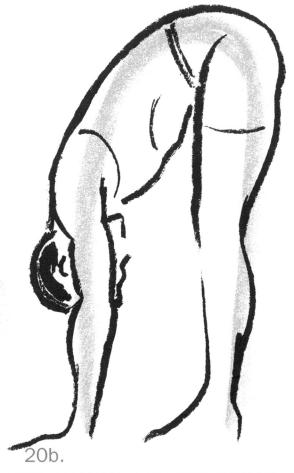

20b.

21.

Legs together squats with jumps

End the starting position of legs together squat with a jump into the air, raising hands overhead. Return to starting position.

Reps: beginning 2–4
intermediate 6
advanced 10

Sets: 3

Weights: None

22a.   22b.

22.
Half-squats with jumps
Squat from halfway down, without putting hands on floor, and jump, then return to squat.
Reps: beginning 2–4
     intermediate 6
     advanced 10
Sets: 3
Weights: None

23.
Basketball jumps
Stand, hands in front of chest as if holding a basketball. Bend your knees and spring up, lifting both arms into the air as if shooting the ball. Land softly, allowing your knees to bend again, and jump back up. Shake legs and rest for 20 to 30 seconds after each sequence.
Reps: beginning 4
     intermediate 6–8
     advanced 10
Sets: 3
Weights: None

24.
Lunge scissors
Lunge deeply with your left leg forward, then switch legs, by pushing off into a light jump so that the right leg is in front. Scissor legs in a continuous motion. Can be executed with a small pause as you return to starting position. Rest 20 to 30 seconds after completing all sets of lunge scissors, lunge twists, and side-to-side skating.
Reps: beginning 4
     intermediate 6
     advanced 10
Sets: 3
Weights: None

25.
Lunge twists
Assume lunge position and place your hands on your hips, keeping your body straight. Jump up and turn in the air so that you land with your left knee bent and your right leg extended behind you. Continue jumping and twisting without pausing, making sure that your legs, not your back, take the landing shock. Can be executed with a small pause as you switch lunges.
Reps: beginning 4
     intermediate 6
     advanced 10
Sets: 3
Weights: None

26.

Side-to-side skating

Cross your right leg behind the left one, extending it far to the side and bending both knees so that you can touch the floor beside your left foot with your right hand. Extend your left arm toward the ceiling. Spring up, changing the position of your body in the air, so that you land with your left leg crossed behind the right, your left hand on the floor beside your right foot, and your right arm extended. Continue switching from side to side in a continuous movement.

Reps: beginning 4
          intermediate 6
          advanced 10
Sets: 3
Weights: None

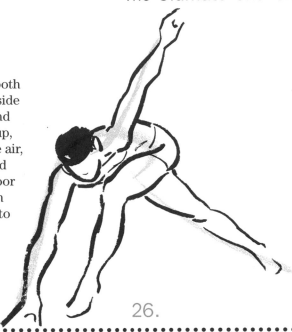

26.

WAIST

Caution: If you have back problems or experience any discomfort while doing these exercises, concentrate on crunches instead. If back problems persist, see a doctor. Aim for a total of 225–300 reps in abdominal exercises. After back extensions with a twist, stretch the full length of your body while still on your back. Bring your knees to your chest and wrap your arms around your shins, chin to chest; rock back and forth 4 to 10 times.

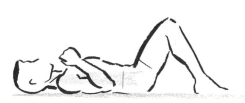

27a.

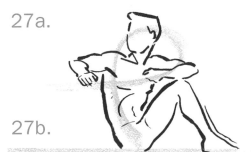

27b.

27.

Sit-ups with twist

Lie on your back, knees bent, feet apart. Bend your elbows close to your sides, hands lightly fisted. Roll up, contracting your abdominal muscles and twist your torso to the right, bringing your arms parallel to the floor. Straighten your torso before returning to start. Your shoulders should touch the floor. Complete all reps to right before switching to left.

Reps: beginning 4
          intermediate 6
          advanced 25 or more
Sets: 2–4 each side
Weights: None

28.

Pendulums

Lie on your back, arms to sides, legs together and extended toward ceiling. Controlling the movement, lower—do not drop—both legs to the right, without letting your back come off the floor. Lift both legs to ceiling, then lower them to the other side. Keep in mind that the straighter your legs, the more difficult the move, so start with legs bent and progress to straighter legs. You may also wish to put a pillow under your head for support.

Reps: beginning 4
        intermediate 6
        advanced 25 or more
Sets: 2–4 each side
Weights: None

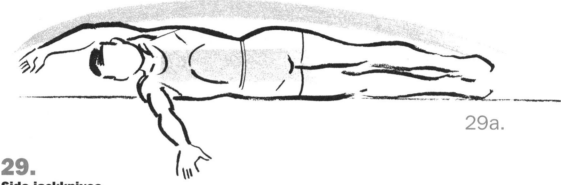

29a.

29.

Side jackknives

Lie on your right side, legs straight, the left one "stacked" directly on top of the right. Extend your right arm straight in front of you on the floor, palm down, and bring your left arm slightly behind your head. Lift both legs toward the ceiling (they will naturally move forward) while pushing on floor with right hand. At the same time lift your torso and reach toward your toes with your left arm. Use your right arm for support.

Reps: beginning 4
        intermediate 6
        advanced 25 or more
Sets: 2–4 each side
Weights: None

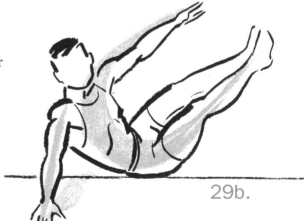

29b.

30.

Back extensions

Standing with feet wide apart and knees slightly bent, bend your torso toward your toes, allowing your arms to relax down toward the floor. Stand up tall, reaching your arms toward the ceiling, then bend forward and down again in a continuous movement. Rest 10 to 15 seconds and begin again.

Reps: beginning 4
          intermediate 6
          advanced 10

Sets: 2–3

Weights: None; as this exercise becomes easier, add 5-, 8-, or 10-lb. dumbbells

30a.   30b.

31.

Back extensions with twist

Standing with legs wide and slightly bent, bend down toward the right and touch your toes with both hands. Stand up, twisting to face left and reaching toward the ceiling. Allow your right leg to turn with your torso and your right heel to come off the ground. Return to start in a continuous movement. Rest 10 seconds and begin again.

Reps: beginning 4
          intermediate 6
          advanced 10

Sets: 2–3

Weights: None; as this exercise becomes easier, add 5-, 8-, or 10-lb. dumbbells

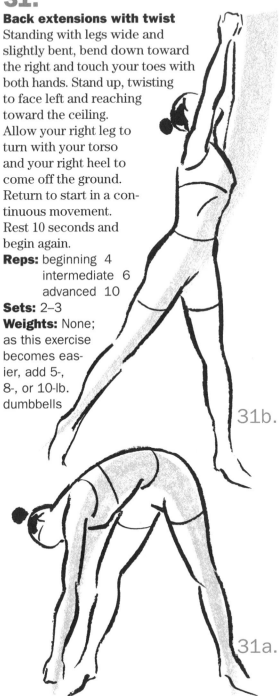

31b.

31a.

ARMS AND CHEST

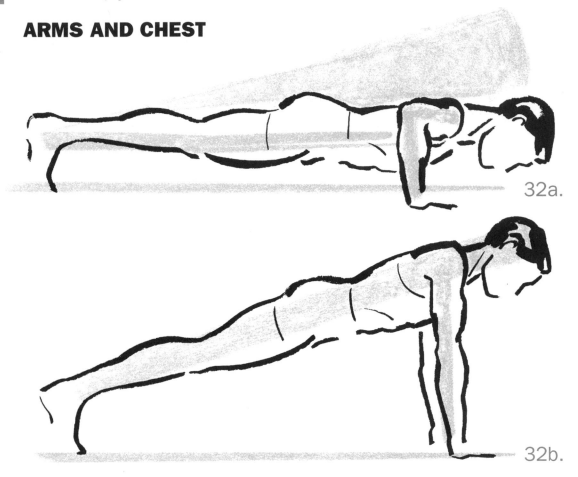

32a.

32b.

32.
Push-ups

Standard: Place your hands on the floor about shoulder-width apart, fingers pointing forward. Extend your legs behind you, feet together and balanced on toes. Make sure your head is in line with your spine. Tighten your abs and lower back and tuck your pelvis so that your body is straight (no arching). Keeping your body stiff as a board, bend your elbows until your chest is just a few inches from the floor, then return to starting position.

Modified: Kneel on hands and knees, hands shoulder-width apart, fingers facing forward. Bring your feet off the floor, tuck your pelvis, and tighten your knees. Bend your elbows until your chest is just a few inches from the floor, then return to starting position. Exhale as you push up and inhale as you go down.

Reps: beginning 8
intermediate 10
advanced 25 or more

Sets: 3

Weights: None

33.

Wide-arm push-ups
Assume the standard push-ups position, only this time separate your hands a bit wider than shoulder distance apart, the fingers pointing out on a diagonal.
Reps: beginning 4
        intermediate 6
        advanced 10
Sets: 3
Weights: None

34.

Hands-together push-ups
Assume the standard push-ups position, but keep hands right under your chest, fingers pointing in and touching, elbows out to the sides.
Reps: beginning 4
        intermediate 6
        advanced 10
Sets: 3
Weights: None

WEIGHTS

If you feel any discomfort in your shoulders, adjust the angle or amount of weight until comfortable. If discomfort persists, disregard these exercises.
Complete three rotations of the bench presses, lateral flyes, and pullovers, resting for 10 seconds after each rotation.

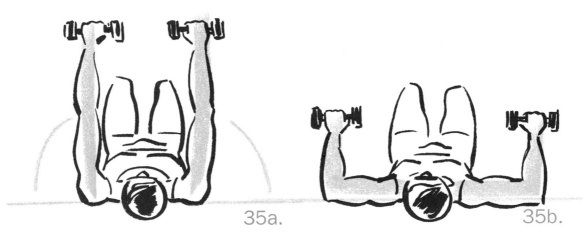

35a. 35b.

35.

Bench presses
Lie on your back, knees bent, holding a dumbbell in each hand. Extend both arms toward the ceiling, palms facing forward. Bring elbows toward the floor, then straighten arms back toward ceiling.

Reps: beginning 4
        intermediate 6
        advanced 10
Sets: 3
Weights: Women 5–10 lbs.
           Men 10–20 lbs.

36.

Lateral flyes

Face palms in and bend elbows slightly. Inhaling, open both arms wide to the sides as far as you can, feeling a stretch across your chest. Exhale and return to starting position, contracting your chest as you bring the dumbbells together.

Reps: beginning 4
        intermediate 6
        advanced 10

Sets: 3

Weights: Women 5–10 lbs.
           Men 10–20 lbs.

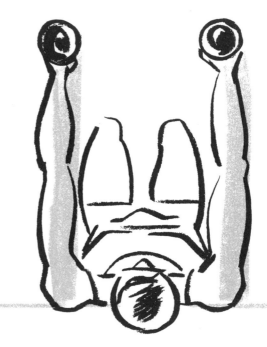

36a.

36b.

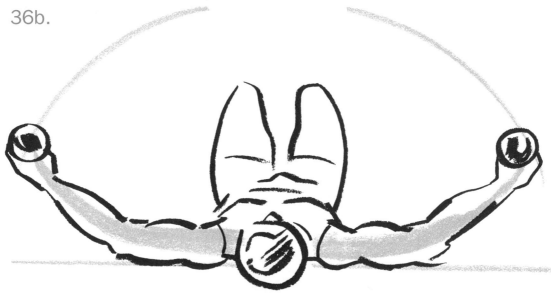

37.

Pullovers

Face knuckles in and close
together, bend elbows
slightly. Inhaling, bring both
arms over your head as far
as you can, tapping weights
lightly on the floor, then
exhale and bring them back
to starting position.

Reps: beginning 4
intermediate 6
advanced 10

Sets: 3

Weights: Women 5–10 lbs.
Men 10–20 lbs.

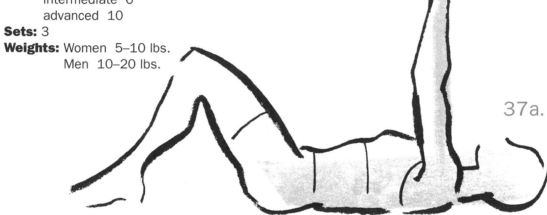

37a.

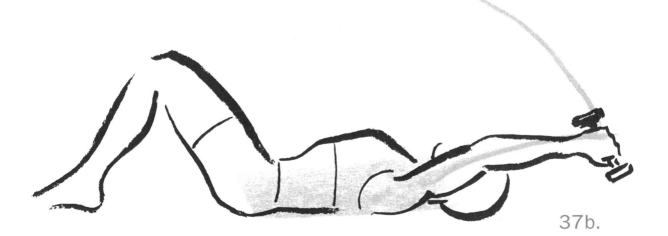

37b.

Complete three rotations of alternating reverse curls, behind-the-neck triceps extensions, breast strokes, bent-over rows, and side bends, which serve as rest.

38.

Alternating reverse curls
Stand, feet shoulder-width apart, knees slightly bent. Grasp a dumbbell in each hand, pal— Lock you— your ribs for the entire exercise. Alternate bringing the weight to each shoulder in a continuous motion; time breathing to either arm's curls.

Reps: beginning 4
intermediate 6
advanced 10
Sets: 3
Weights: Women 5–10 lbs.
Men 10–20 lbs.

39.

Behind-the-neck triceps extensions
Stand, feet shoulder-width apart, knees slightly bent. Grasp the top of a dumbbell with both hands and hold it behind your head, elbows pointing up and upper arms close to your head. Straighten arms to lift weight toward ceiling without moving upper arms, then return to starting position. Exhale as you lift the dumbbell up, inhale as you lower it.
Reps: beginning 4
intermediate 6
advanced 10
Sets: 3
Weights: Women 5–10 lbs.
Men 10–20 lbs.

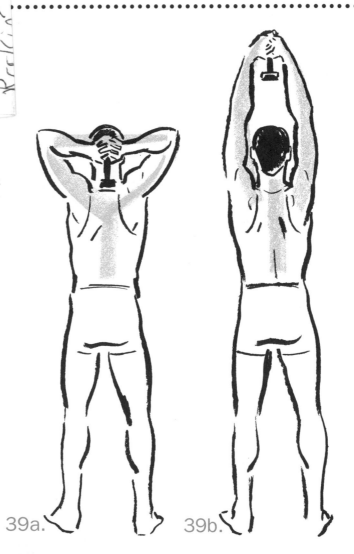

39a.   39b.

40.

Breast strokes

Holding a dumbbell in each hand, extend arms in front of you, fingers pointing down. Maintain a low center of gravity and use your hips to balance you. In a continuous movement, imitate the breast stroke from swimming, keeping your elbows up as you pull weights toward you and letting them drop as you bring them along your torso to prepare to push out again. Continue moving weights in front of you and to your sides without stopping until you have completed a full set of reps.

Reps: beginning 4
          intermediate 6
          advanced 10
Sets: 3
Weights: Women 5–10 lbs.
         Men 10–20 lbs.

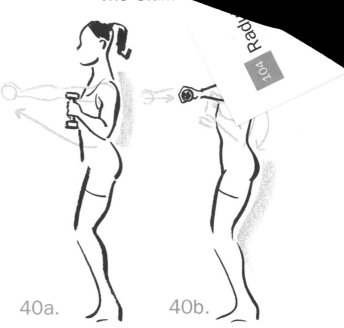

40a.   40b.

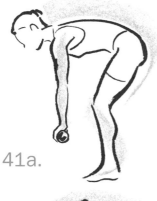

41a.

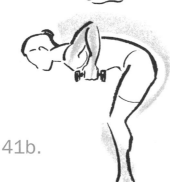

41b.

41.

Bent-over rows

Holding a dumbbell in each hand, bend forward and extend both arms toward the floor, palms facing your shins. Bend your elbows toward the ceiling and *pull* weight to chest level, working against gravity.

Reps: beginning 4
          intermediate 6
          advanced 10
Sets: 3
Weights: Women 5–10 lbs.
         Men 10–20 lbs.

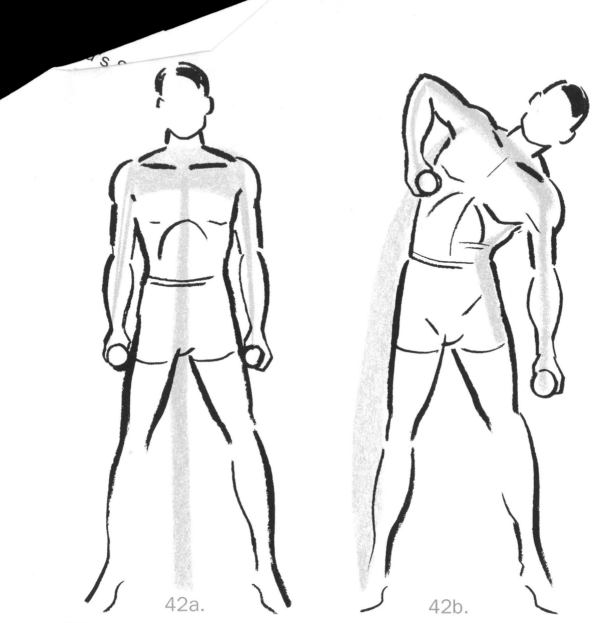

42a.

42b.

42.

Side bends

Stand, feet slightly more than shoulder-width apart, knees slightly bent. Hold a dumbbell in each hand, arms at sides. Bend your torso to the left, bringing your right elbow toward the ceiling, then return to start. Complete 1 set on right side before starting on left side, then switch for remaining sets.

Reps: beginning 4
intermediate 6
advanced 10

Sets: 3

Weights: Women 5–10 lbs.
Men 10–20 lbs.

Complete three rotations of squat curls, behind-the-back lateral raises, overhead presses with a twist, and side bends, which serve as rest.

43.

Squat curls

Squat, feet pointing slightly outward, thighs parallel to floor. Do not let knees extend past toes. Grasp a dumbbell in each hand and extend arms straight toward floor, palms facing out. Arms should not rest on thigh. Bring weights to shoulder height, then lower them slowly, resisting the pull of gravity.

Reps: beginning 4
intermediate 6
advanced 10
Sets: 3
Weights: Women 5–10 lbs.
Men 10–20 lbs.

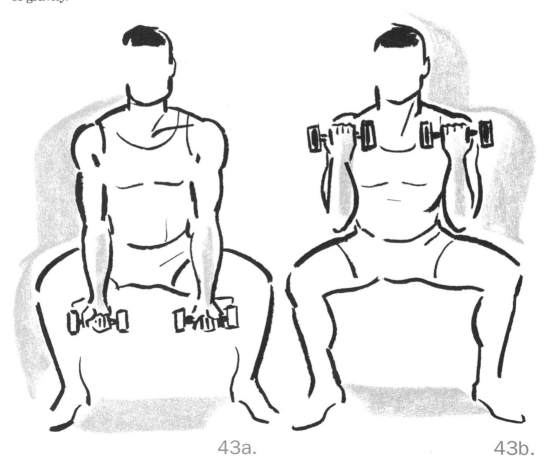

43a.   43b.

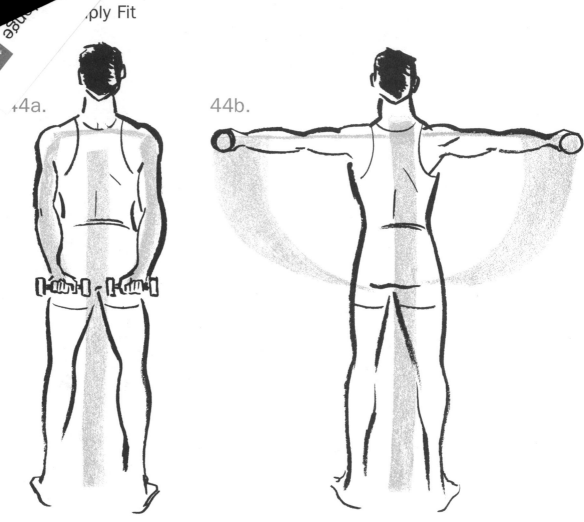

44a.

44b.

44.

Behind-the-back lateral raises

Stand, feet shoulder-width apart, knees
slightly bent. Grasp a dumbbell in each hand
behind back, arms straight and palms facing
away from body. Raise arms to the sides to
shoulder height, turning them slightly so
that palms face down. Keep shoulders
relaxed; don't allow them to bunch up
toward ears. Keep elbows slightly bent.

Reps: beginning 4
       intermediate 6
       advanced 10
Sets: 3
Weights: Women 5–10 lbs.
       Men 10–20 lbs.

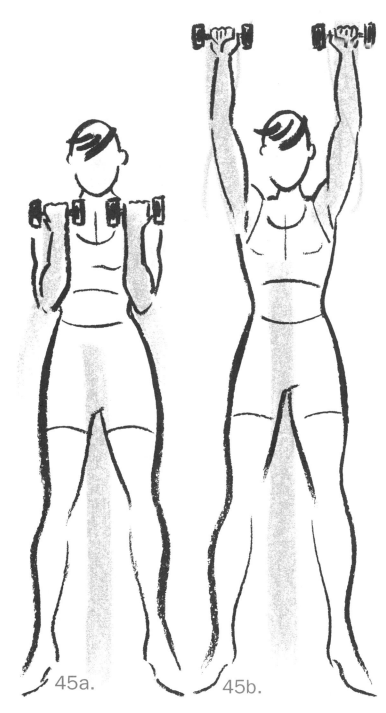

45a.

45b.

45.

Overhead presses with a twist

Stand with feet comfortably apart, knees relaxed. Hold a dumbbell in each hand at shoulder-level, elbows pointing down, fingers facing you. Exhale and bring arms straight up toward ceiling, while at the same time turning your hands so the fingers are facing out. As you inhale, return weights to shoulders, turning hands to face you. Be careful not to snap your elbow into place as you lift. Also try to press faster than you lower the weights.

Reps: beginning 4
        intermediate 6
        advanced 10

Sets: 3

Weights: Women 5–10 lbs.
          Men 10–20 lbs.

46.

Side bends

See page 104 for description. Rest for 15–30 seconds.

Reps: beginning 4
        intermediate 6
        advanced 10

Sets: 3

Weights: Women 5–10 lbs.
          Men 10–20 lbs.

three rotations of alternating upright rows, sun fists, and side bends,
erve as rest.

Alternating upright rows

Stand, feet shoulder-width
apart, knees slightly bent.
Hold a dumbbell in each
hand at thigh level. Leading
with your elbow, lift the
weight in your right hand to
shoulder level. As you lower
it, repeat the move with your
left arm. Continue, alternating sides. Time your breathing to either arm's row.

Reps: beginning 4
intermediate 6
advanced 10

Sets: 3

Weights: Women 5–10 lbs.
Men 10–20 lbs.

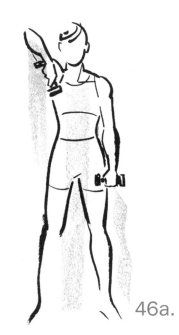
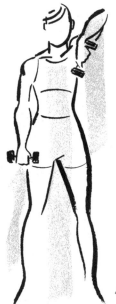

46a. 46b.

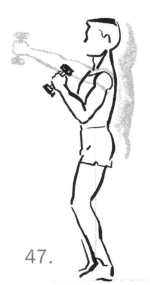

47.

47.

Sun fists

Stand, feet shoulder-width
apart, knees slightly bent,
abdominals and hips tight.
Hold dumbbells in each hand at
chest level, palms facing each
other. Punch your right arm
forward and slightly toward
ceiling in a fluid motion, without locking your elbow. Then
bring it back as you punch your
left arm forward and up.
Continue, alternating sides.

Reps: beginning 4
intermediate 6
advanced 10

Sets: 3

Weights: Women 5–10 lbs.
Men 10–20 lbs.

48.

Side bends

See page 104 for description.
Rest for 15–30 seconds.

Reps: beginning 4
intermediate 6
advanced 10

Sets: 3

Weights: Women 5–10 lbs.
Men 10–20 lbs.

Complete three rotations of alternating regular curls, alternating overhead presses, and side bends, which serve as rest.

49.

Alternating regular curls

Stand, feet shoulder-width apart, knees slightly bent and hips tight. Hold your arms at your sides, keeping your elbows locked against ribcage and your palms facing upward.

Without moving upper arms, alternate bending each elbow to bring the weights to your shoulders. Time breathing to either arm's curl and continue, alternating sides.

Reps: beginning 4
       intermediate 6
       advanced 10
Sets: 3
Weights: Women 5–10 lbs.
        Men 10–20 lbs.

50a.

50b.

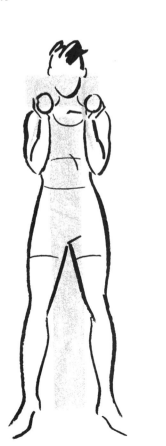
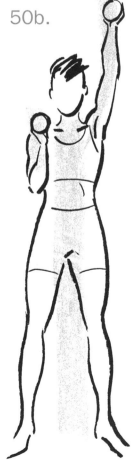

50.

Alternating overhead presses

Stand, feet shoulder-width apart, knees slightly bent. Hold a dumbbell in each hand at shoulder level, fingers facing in, elbows pointing down. Alternate pressing each weight straight up toward the ceiling. Time breathing to either arm's press and continue alternating.

Reps: beginning 4
       intermediate 6
       advanced 10
Sets: 3
Weights: Women 5–10 lbs.
        Men 10–20 lbs.

51.

Side bends

See page 104 for description. Rest for 15–30 seconds.

Reps: beginning 4
       intermediate 6
       advanced 10
Sets: 3
Weights: Women 5–10 lbs.
        Men 10–20 lbs.

Complete ten rotations of wrist curls and reverse wrist curls, resting for 10–30 seconds after each rotation.

52.

Wrist curls (on chair)

Kneeling, position both arms across the seat of a chair, a dumbbell in each hand, palms facing up. Moving only your wrists, curl the weights toward you, then lower them to starting position.

Reps: beginning 4
        intermediate 6
        advanced 10

Sets: 10

Weights: Women 5–10 lbs.
          Men 10–20 lbs.

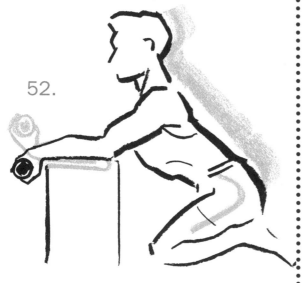

53.

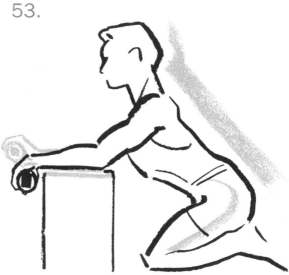

53.

Reverse wrist curls (on chair)

Kneel beside a chair as for wrist curls, this time with palms facing down. Curl weights up, again moving only your wrists, then return to starting position.

Reps: beginning 4
        intermediate 6
        advanced 10

Sets: 10

Weights: Women 5–10 lbs.
          Men 10–20 lbs.

COOL DOWN

STRETCHES

54.

Straddle

Sit up straight, legs as wide apart as is comfortable, feet flexed. Raise both arms overhead. Stretch forward at the hips as far as you can, being careful not to bend at the waist. Don't worry if you can only go a few inches; the point is to feel a stretch along your inner thighs. Stretch to left toe; to right toe; to middle.

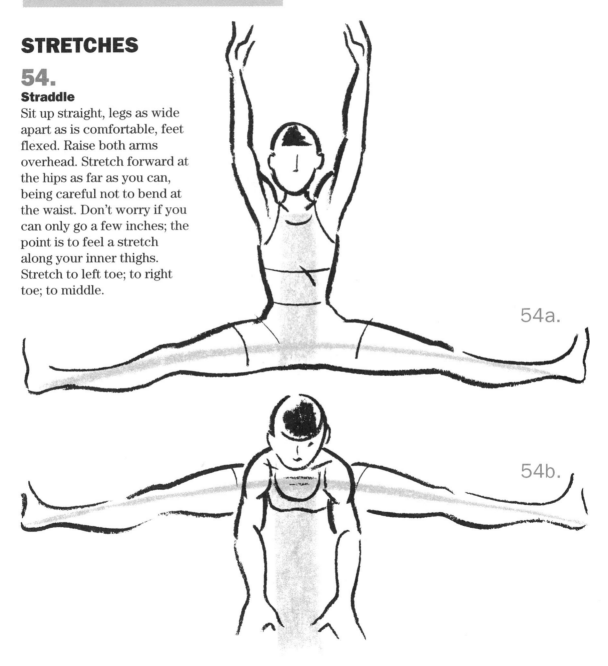

54a.

54b.

55.
Side-to-side
Maintain position and bend sideways to the left, stretching your right arm over your head. Switch to other side. Hold for 10 seconds, count to 12.

56.
Half-diamond
Sit up with your right leg extended at a slight angle, your left leg bent so that your foot is tucked against your right upper thigh; stretch your torso over your right leg, reaching for your toes; hold, then switch legs.

57.
Diamond
Sit up straight and bring your feet toward you, soles together. Use your hands to gently pull your feet closer, pressing down with your knees so that you feel a stretch all along your inner thighs. Hold for 10 seconds, count to 12.

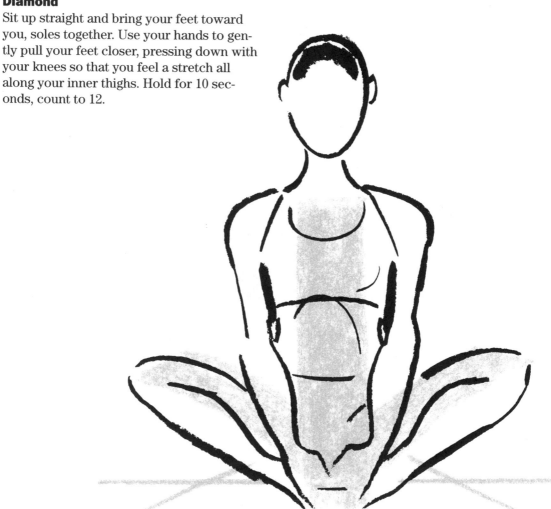

57.

58.

Doorjamb

Place your right palm against a doorjamb or column, right arm straight out to your side and parallel to floor. Step forward with your right foot to turn your body toward the left. You should feel a stretch along the length of your right arm, extending to the right side of your chest. Hold, then repeat with left hand.

59.

Quads

Stand with your right hand against a wall or chair for support. Bend your left leg and grasp the ankle with your left hand; gently pull your heel toward your buttocks, keeping your pelvis tucked to prevent your back from arching, and to get the most effective stretch. Hold each for 10 seconds, count to 12.

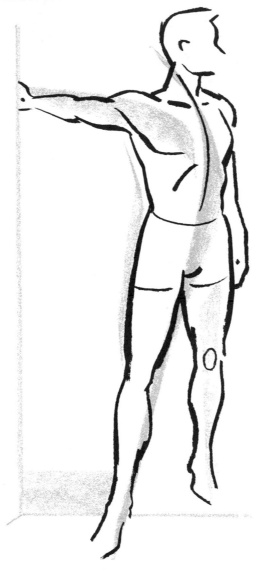

58.

The Outdoor Gym

Somewhere along the line, the modern fitness boom has made people think that they have to go indoors to exercise; that somehow the beauty and diversity of the world outdoors is too distracting and too unstructured. The health club mentality has put blinders on us all—myself included for a while—and made us believe that getting healthy and strengthening our bodies is something that has to happen indoors. I guess that people think that exercise is medicine, and it has to taste like medicine.

All I have to do is point this out to you, and I think you see what a limiting attitude it is. And you probably recognize how boxed in you have become in your own attitude toward what constitutes exercise. If it helps, look at the outdoors as another wide-open gym, ready for you to join.

This chapter is about helping you break out of the box; both the physical box in which you are exercising, and the mental box that has locked you inside a room. The world is waiting just outside the window.

Recently, one of the hottest "gyms" in New York has been a facility called the Chelsea Piers. Some smart developers took over a group of huge abandoned piers on the Hudson River and converted them into a group of oversize recreational playgrounds for adults: they have an Olympic-size pool, a "mountain" for climbing, a field for playing soccer, a simulated driving range, and much more. Everyone is very excited about having all of these facilities together, particularly since New York City is starved for recreational activities. But New Yorkers are also starved for the latest thing, and everybody nowadays likes the superstore concept of packing everything under one roof.

I'm all for facilities like this, but I also like to point out to people that there's another great multifaceted health facility like this right near my home in Scarsdale: it's called Westchester County. We have cliffs to climb, trails to ski and bike on, fields to play on, a beautiful river for kayaking, and much more. Best of all, the facilities are free and they are rarely crowded. I bet you have a great facility just like this near your home too.

I've always known, and underscored, that training in the gym is nothing but preparation for and a supplement to natural movement, whether natural movement means washing your car and lugging around groceries, or running around the park and blading around the neighborhood. The point of my program is to use the gym to prepare within the confines of a safe and controlled environment for the real world outside our doors. Even a gym like mine, which is constructed to help perform natural activities like running, skipping, throwing, and climbing, still can't duplicate the multitude of conditions nor the enormous spaces of the outdoors.

As I discovered when I had my epiphany in training Bianca Jagger, you can actually make a gym for yourself outside, bringing some of the carefully constructed programming of what happens in the gym to the most natural place of all for training—outdoors. The basic Class, the Personal Training exercises, and the Ultimate Challenge will have already laid the base for taking your training outside.

As we all know, elite athletes train outdoors regularly, where they are forced to solve the obsta-cles Mother Nature sets up for them. They run in sand and up and down hills, slalom around trees, climb down embankments, leap over fallen logs. These athletes understand that success comes from breaking the cycle of training and varying the routine as much as possible. By walking out your door, you do the same. When you exercise outside, the sky literally is your only limit.

Even if you first venture outside to run or swim or cycle because you know these activities are good for your body, I guarantee you will soon get caught up in the glory of being outdoors and moving within that environment. In the mid-1970s, I used to bike in Central Park with an informal group, but after a while we wanted to expand our horizons. We bought fancier all-terrain bikes and began taking trips out of the city. The first time I took a group to East Hampton, more than a hundred miles, I didn't really know the Long Island area all that well, so it was an adventure for all of us. It was amazing that with the exception of a few flat tires, we made it. It took us about six hours, and most of my fellow cyclists would never have believed that they could complete a

Do something different every day.

Playing is no fun if you are not ready.

who can climb the highest, run the fastest, score the most baskets, ace every serve. But for grown-ups, it's about teamwork. If you're playing a game, other players will love teaching you as much as competing against you. Think about Regis, ribbing poor Boris about his basketball playing—but he was teaching him as well. Having someone to share the experience makes it all the richer and provides an encouraging accomplice, ready to help get you back out there again.

trip like that. What a thrill it was to see the amazement on their faces. Our destination was the home of a friend who had a pool, and I can still remember the feeling of jumping in with my clothes on, exhausted and ecstatic.

There was no stopping us after that. We would go out on weekends and ride for hours. Soon we began carrying backpacks and tents with us so we could stay overnight. At the end of each journey, inevitably someone would say, "I never dreamed I could do what I just did. Now I know what I'm really capable of."

You never know how much you can do until you try. Still, it can be intimidating to face the challenges of the world outside. You feel small, especially if you are used to working out in front of a mirror, where your reality is reduced to the tiny world of you and your reflection. That's okay: fear teaches respect and humility. Use that humility when you first venture outdoors, and you will be fine. The trick is to let Mother Nature teach you, to join forces with her, and to take things at a reasonable pace.

Don't go it alone. With children and teenagers, sports are all about competition:

The other great thing about the outdoors is that it's never too late to start, and the obstacles to getting going are minimal. Today's walker is tomorrow's cyclist or runner. You can start at any age, and you can start as modestly or ambitiously as is appropriate. No matter what you are doing, you will reap the immediate benefits of enjoying the outdoors and the sensation of using your body again.

Charlie, a director of liver transplants at a major New York hospital and a dear friend, was wary of sports and athletics because he was overweight and sedentary. For weeks I tried to get him out in a kayak. "Not for me," he'd say. "I'm too big." One afternoon I stopped by his house in Montauk, Long Island, after kayaking with some of my students from the gym, and I told him all about it. And then it came out: "Radu," he said, "I really wish I had the courage to do this."

Ah! My chance. We got into my double kayak so he wouldn't feel nervous about being on the water alone, and we went into the ocean right then and there. That's all it took to hook Charlie. He was amazed at how it made him feel. "This is such a transcendence," he told me. Now Charlie has two kayaks, and he goes with his family all the time. He even bought a four-wheel-drive car so he could transport the kayaks, and is dreaming of a kayaking trip in the British Virgin Islands.

If you have been away from activity for a long time, like Charlie, you may not be as sure of your abilities. Somewhere along the line we get the idea into our heads that there is nothing we can do to stop the decline of our bodies. We resign ourselves to a sedentary lifestyle, and hope to at least keep our wits about us as long as possible. Realistically, everything becomes harder as we get older, whether it's getting down the stairs in the morning or getting ourselves to swim those laps. It's the oldest principle of physics—a body in motion tends to stay in motion, and a body at rest tends to stay at rest.

The first step, out of the chair and onto your feet, is always the hardest one. But the benefits of regular exercise are actually greater for those of you who are getting on in years—not so much because you'll live longer, which is what your doctor will tell you, but because you'll live better.

The people who stay happiest as they grow older are the ones who maintain their appetite for all aspects of life. Your body isn't just a vessel for carting around your brain. The two work in inextricable tandem.

Let me assure you, as long as you're realistic about it, you can jump into the game at any time. Just look at me—I'm living proof that a short Romanian guy in his

early fifties can run the pants off just about anybody out there. Of course this is both my profession and my passion, but the point is that there is nothing unique about me and my physical capabilities. I do the work and I reap the rewards, and I can assure you that I plan on training people and enjoying being active for the rest of my days. I can't imagine life any other way, and once you realize that age is no obstacle, you too will refuse to allow yourself to become a victim of gravity and inertia. As I told you in the introduction, the key to fitness isn't physical, it's mental. It's all about your attitude about what is possible. Once you believe that you can use your body again, that you must do so, then the rest will flow naturally.

Sure, you probably can't run as fast, jump as high, swing a bat as hard, or throw a ball as far as you did in the eleventh grade. But even professional athletes slow down.

In our lives, there is no stopping, only regressing. Stopping means death.

They set up friendly reunion matches on weekends and get people together for touch football, doubles tennis, or to shoot some hoops. They don't park, they just move into a slower lane, or they get on a different road and pick up outdoor sports like hiking, canoeing, swimming, or mountaineering that keep them in shape without aggravating old injuries.

Actually, my friend Charlie is typical of a lot of the baby boomers who come to my gym. These people are accomplished achievers in almost all facets of their lives. Even though they may not have exercised or done anything physical in years, their spirit of adventure is an engine awaiting the initial spark. They are doers, and once they decide to get active again, they can't wait for the fun part. They want to jump in a kayak, or wheel around on a fancy mountain bike, or zoom down the slopes.

I want you to become passionate about activity as well, regardless of your age, but love only grows from an open mind. If you take up a sport simply because you've heard it's a great cardiovascular workout, you're missing the boat. There's danger in exercising simply for cosmetic reasons, or to improve your health. Activity becomes bitter medicine needed to prevent death. Not only that, but you get too concerned about the numbers: the repetitions, the miles logged, the pounds lost, the heartbeats per minute. A beautiful and joyful activity becomes just another dehumanizing set of statistics.

Ultimately, you shortchange yourself by being too single-minded. In the outdoor gym, the first rule is to open your eyes and look around you. Stop being focused on your body, and start being focused on your world—that's where the real payoff lies. The first time I went kayaking with Michael Gelman, the executive producer for *Live with Regis and Kathie Lee*, we went to Sag Harbor, New York. I taught him how to paddle on shore, and then we hit the water. He was in terrific shape already, but after about twenty minutes he was exhausted, and raving, "Man, this is great cardiovascular work!" My response was, "Yeah, but did you see those seals on the rocks over there?" When he looked up and saw these beautiful wild creatures so close and in their natural habitat, he exclaimed, "Oh, my God. Unbelievable!" Once he looked beyond his inner world, he saw the real reward of kayaking.

Just as you want to round out your perspective, ideally you want to round out your exercise program with a variety of outdoor sports. This will work your muscles and your mind in a variety of ways, so there's less danger that you will become bored or will injure yourself by overusing a specific body part and underusing others. The best way is to pick two or three sports that you enjoy, but which offer benefits that will work together to build

Sprint on your bike. Challenge a hill.

overall fitness. Racquetball and golf, for instance, are very different in competitive terms, but they are both unilateral sports: they use one side of the upper body more than the other. So you would need to combine them with an activity like swimming, in which you can vary your stroke and give both sides of your body equal attention. As another example, you could balance the terrific lower-body benefits of cycling with something like basketball or tennis. In addition to working your arms and shoulders, these sports will challenge your lower body in a different way, by requiring you to move sideways, backward, and even vertically as you jump up to shoot a basket or reach for a sky-high return. With combinations like these, you can turn a single Saturday adventure into a cross-training dream.

The following is a guide to nineteen popular sports and outdoor activities, to help you take what you like to do and do it better, and in a way that's good for your overall fitness. Each description identifies the main physical benefits of the given activity and offers a short tip on how to help prepare yourself for maximum performance. Additionally, I've given you suggestions for little twists that will help expand a straightforward sport, like basketball, into a more complete and more balanced workout that will help prepare you for any physical challenges. With each of these activities, be sure to prepare yourself with the proper equipment, safety instructions, stretches, and lessons, if necessary.

You are already the king of your house— now see if you measure up in the world. Go outside.

TIPS FOR 19 POPULAR ACTIVITIES
Below are six activities that are great for leg and lower-body exercise—and a smart way to start exercising outdoors.

Power Walking
Lower-body strength, aerobic endurance.

Take very long steps forward for one minute, then take giant steps backward for fifteen to thirty seconds. Do as many sets as you can; repeat as often as you like during your walk, exaggerating your hip movement. Because your arms and shoulders tend to get tired, shore up their strength by strapping on wrist weights. You may also choose to run, walk backward, or stride sideways, crossing one leg over the other.

Hiking
Cardiovascular endurance, leg strength, sense of direction.

Fill your backpack with books and strap it on during your evening power walks. Keep adding books as the load begins to seem lighter, and wear your hiking boots to break them in. Jump from high to low benches to learn to land softly and firmly. Carry a stick while training for hikes. The average length of a half-day hike is 7–10 miles; 12–20 miles for a full day.

Mountaineering and Climbing
Aerobic conditioning, balance and coordination, total body strengthening, powers of concentration, courage.

To increase the gripping power of your fingers on rocks, hang from a chin-up bar or edge of a doorway by all eight fingers; one at a time, lift up your pinkies, then your ring fingers. Clamber over obstacles, like medicine balls, or anything you come upon for balance. Also climb ropes, hike, and do lots of push-ups and pull-ups.

Cycling (Touring)
Stamina, lower-body strength.

Start with lower gears to promote spinning and then shift to higher gears to make the work harder and promote strength. Break rhythm and do interval training or fartlek training.

Mountain Biking
Lower-body strength and upper-body strength, agility, balance.

In a flat, traffic-free area, such as an empty parking lot, do each of the following: Cycle in a slalom pattern from one end of the lot to the other; circle to the left six to ten times, starting with very wide circles and gradually making them tighter; repeat to the right; do six to ten figure eights, then six to ten tiny wheelies, lifting the front of the bike up a few inches, as if hopping over a stick or stone in your path. Finish by practicing mounting and dismounting the bike in slow motion.

In-Line Skating
Lower-body strength, endurance, balance.

Walk and run on grass while wearing skates. Also practice skating in circles, bringing your heels together and bending your knees, and skating in figure eights. The plié squats in Personal Training (page 61) are great for stretching and building the muscles used in in-line skating.

Here are five activities which provide good upper-body strength; some incorporate total body conditioning, too.

Swimming

Total body strength, stamina.

Do one lap using only your legs (using a kickboard), one lap using only your right arm (freestyle), one lap using only the left arm. Repeat this sequence four to six times. For deck training, use pulleys and rubber bands while practicing various strokes to get the feel of the water's resistance.

Kayaking

Upper body and midsection strength, cardiovascular endurance, balance and coordination, speed of reaction.

Do ten to twenty strokes of the following in a kayak: Lean to the right, then lean to the left, then row backward; finally do six to ten or more figure eights. Try the broomstick twist from Personal Training (page 65) and modify it by bending side to side.

Rowing

Total body strength (upper body is mostly pulling, and legs are pushing and pulling), stamina.

Do each of the following for ten to twenty strokes: Row, emphasizing the work of your legs; then arms; then back. Next, combine using only your legs and back, then your arms and back, then your legs and arms. The bent-over row exercises from the Class (page 35) work the arm and chest muscles used for rowing also.

Cross-Country Skiing

Total body strengthening, aerobic stamina.

Repeat this sequence ten to twenty times: Take two "steps" forward, left then right, then bring both poles forward, dig in, and push. Repeat, left, right, and *push*. When you've completed one set, repeat, this time ending with three pushes in succession (left, right, push, push, push; left, right, push, push, push); again, do ten to twenty. Concentrate on squats and back extensions from earlier chapters to prepare.

Downhill Skiing

Upper- and lower-body strength, balance and coordination, speed of execution, speed of reaction.

Scissor your legs rapidly into deep lunges to improve balance and strength. In the off-season, run down a wooded hill, slaloming between the trees.

The following popular sports involve strategy and overall physical ability, and, for most, teamwork.

Golf

Torso flexibility, hand-eye coordination, concentration.

Stretch with a club: Hold it behind your neck and twist to the left and right, ten to twenty times. Place the club on the ground, handle side up; wrap both hands around the handle, and bend forward at the hips until you feel a stretch in your lower back; hold for a count of twelve. Hold a club at both ends and bring your arms straight overhead and behind you as far as you can; hold for a count of twelve.

Tennis

Lower-body stamina, strength, speed of reaction and speed of execution, hand-eye coordination, multidirectional movement, strategic thinking.

Standing beside and a few yards away from a partner, toss a ball, preferably a medicine ball, back and forth. Use both hands, keeping the arms straight. Sprint court lines and add a side lunge to replicate stretching for hard-to-reach shots.

Basketball

Strength, endurance, speed of all kinds, vertical lift, multidirectional movement, shoulder strength, hand-eye coordination, strategic thinking.

Stand in front of the net, squat, and jump up to try to touch the rim. Do ten or twenty times in succession. If you're on an official court, add sweet-sixteen sprints: sprint from sideline to sideline, bending to touch each one, as fast as you can, sixteen times. Sit in front of a net and try to make baskets. Try this from various points in front of and beside the net.

Volleyball

Strength, endurance, speed of all kinds, vertical lift, multidirectional movement, shoulder strength, hand-eye coordination, strategic thinking.

With both hands, toss a volleyball straight overhead ten to twenty times in succession; then stand in front of net, do a half-squat and jump up, reaching your arms up and over the net. Repeat ten to twenty times. Also try tossing the volleyball straight overhead, and, without taking your eyes off the ball, squat and touch the ground. Practice criss crosses, ending in either squats or lunges.

Softball/Baseball

Sprinting speed, torso flexibility, throwing and catching ability, hand-eye coordination.

Make five pitches right-handed, then five left-handed. Then do the following sprinting sequence once: Starting at home plate, sprint to first base; then halfway to second, turn quickly and run back to first; go from first all the way to second, from second halfway to third and back; from second all the way to third; from third halfway to home; and finally, from third all the way to home.

Touch Football

Sprinting, quick turning, catching, throwing.

Do the following sprinting exercise six to ten times: Sprint forward ten to twenty yards, turn, and continue running backward ten to twenty yards, turn, and then cut to right for ten yards. Repeat from beginning, cutting to the left. Toss the football in the air a little in front of you and catch it: increase the distance you throw the ball, so that you have to run faster each time.

Soccer

Sprinting speed, agility, speed of reaction, fast thinking.

Sprint ten yards, stop, and jump up. Sashay left ten yards. Sprint ten yards again and jump; sashay right ten yards; repeat the sequence six to ten times. Then dribble the ball between your feet ten to twenty times, then on your knees, then with your head. Kick ball against a wall, first with left foot, then right, using inner and outer part of foot.

Radu-Running
Quadriceps, calves, buttocks, endurance, speed.

Running has become known as an antidote for heart disease, obesity, and other killers. Unfortunately, most runners do it in such a linear and repetitive fashion that they overstress their joints with constant pounding and wind up on the sidelines injured.

Radu-running gives you a thirty-minute heart-jolting jog and will enhance your capability for any sport, while helping to reduce the chance of injury. (However, if you have knee problems, don't attempt this routine without checking with a doctor first.)

Memorize as much of this program as you can and then relax and go out and do as much of it as you can focus on. Don't worry if you skip something, and don't quit, even if you have to slow down or walk. Just keep moving for at least half an hour.

DO THE GENERAL WARM-UP from the Class or the Ultimate Challenge starting on pages 26 and 88, then warm up the muscles that are specific to running using the following stretches:

QUADRICEPS Stand with your right hand against a wall or chair for support. Bend your left leg and grasp the ankle with your left hand; gently pull your heel toward your buttocks, keeping your pelvis tucked to prevent your back from arching, and to get the most effective stretch. Hold for ten seconds (count to twelve), then switch sides.

HAMSTRINGS Cross your left foot over your right and bend forward at the hips as far as you can, reaching your hands toward your toes; you should feel a stretch up the length of both legs. Hold ten seconds (count twelve), cross your right foot over your left, and repeat.

CALVES Stand a little more than arm's length from a wall, feet about hip distance apart. Lean forward and place both hands against the wall; step your right foot back about twelve inches from your left, pressing your heel down toward the floor. Hold ten seconds (count to twelve), then switch sides.

NOW START MOVING, spending one to two minutes on each of the following steps:
1. Begin a normal-paced walk with your arms slightly bent, hands relaxed, swinging gently to the rhythm of your gait.
2. Pick up the pace, taking longer, more determined strides and swinging your arms back and forth from the shoulders.
3. Shorten your stride, moving faster.
4. Begin to run lightly.

COMPLETE THREE ROTATIONS running with knees up, heels to buttocks, followed by light running, and spend about ten seconds on each:
1. Knees up.
2. Heels to buttocks.
3. Light run.

COMPLETE THREE ROTATIONS of light skipping, power skipping, followed by light running, and spend about ten seconds on each:
1. Light skipping.
2. Power skipping (bring knees up high, pump arms from shoulders).
3. Light run.

PERFORM THE FOLLOWING TWO SEGMENTS on flat terrain, so that you can move smoothly and without danger of tripping. Otherwise, skip these and repeat the two rotations above. Complete three rotations of each segment.
1. Run sideways to the right.
2. Run sideways to the left.
3. Criss cross to the right (travel sideways, bringing your left foot in front of your right, then behind your right).
4. Criss cross to the left.
5. Light run.

1. Sashay to the right (moving sideways, take a comfortably wide step to the right, then bring your left foot toward your right, leaping slightly off the ground as they meet). Then sashay to the left.
2. Basketball sashay to the right (move sideways, bending your knees so that you're low to the ground, leading with your right foot and bringing the left to meet it). Basketball sashay to the left.
3. Light run.

CONTINUE RUNNING at whatever pace is comfortable for the duration of your run, taking advantage of whatever obstacles come your way. Jump up to touch the leaves of a tree or to swing from its limbs like a child, leap over a puddle, stop and do some jumping jacks, turn the curb into a balance beam. When you're about five minutes from home, begin to slow down—go from running to light running to power walking to regular walking; don't stop moving until you are breathing normally. Repeat the three stretches above, and treat yourself to plenty of water.

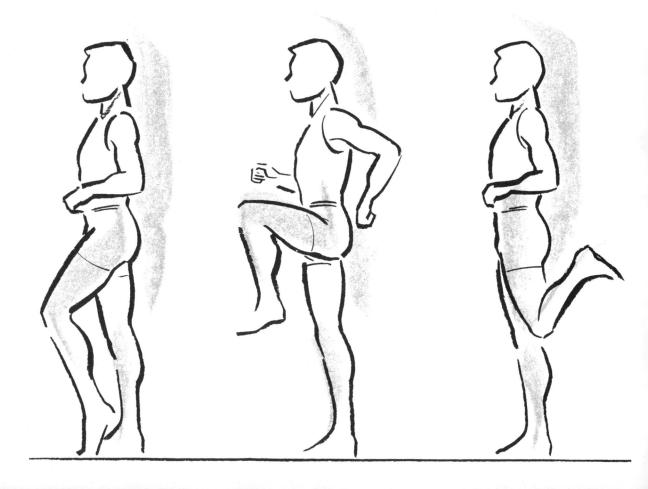

Turning Any Sport into a Training Session

In the first chapter, I discussed how conventional exercise machines are poor training tools because they lead to constant levels of repetitive activity. But when you are out in the real world, everything is variable. You go up and down stairs, around obstacles, speeding up and slowing down, altering your weight load—and that's just getting to work in the morning.

DON'T MAKE THE MISTAKE of transferring bad habits from the indoor gym to the outdoor gym. We all have a tendency to perform at a constant pace; you'll find yourself biking, or skating, or jogging at the same basic pace every time you go out, and before you know it, even the most fun and vigorous activity becomes routine.

WITH INTERVAL TRAINING AND FARTLEK TRAINING, you alternate periods of intense activity with periods of rest or less intense exercise. This is what elite athletes use to maximize their performance; you can apply the same technique to any activity such as swimming, cycling, or rowing. Just follow these general rules for alternating periods of intense activity with more restful ones:
- Begin slowly, in a warm-up phase.
- Move to full sprint speed for a period of 30 to 60 seconds.
- Slow to cruising. Continue modestly until you feel that your heart rate has returned almost to normal and you are not breathing hard. Repeat this cycle five times.
- Go at a comfortable pace for another 2–3 minutes, and cool down and stretch. As you feel you can, increase the distance of your sprinting by 15–30 seconds at a time.

About the author

Radu Teodorescu—well-known as the dean of New York trainers—offers his unique and creative training method at his Physical Culture Studio on West 57th Street in New York City and at his gym in East Hampton, Long Island. In the two decades since he began teaching, Radu's simple, natural style has attracted a steady stream of rave reviews. He has been featured in over 400 magazine articles, and was voted New York City's "Toughest Trainer in Town" by *New York* magazine. In addition, the two award-winning exercise videos Radu created with Cindy Crawford topped the Billboard charts, and the *Cindy Crawford Shape Your Body Workout* was the bestselling fitness tape of all time.

Radu's personal achievements mirror his professional successes. He graduated in 1969 from the Physical Culture University of Bucharest, Romania, after competing since childhood in gymnastics, team handball, soccer, and track and field, on national and international levels.

RADU'S PHYSICAL CULTURE ACTIVEWEAR
Special Limited Edition

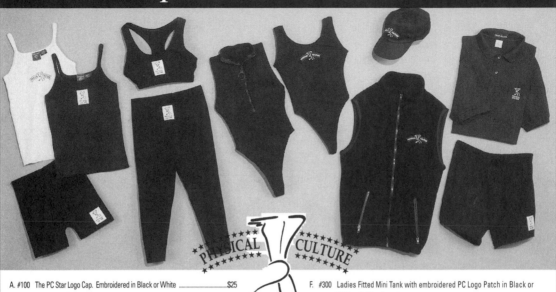

A. **#100** The PC Star Logo Cap. Embroidered in Black or White $25

B. **#200** The Sport Bra with the Logo Patch embroidered on the front, Physical Culture written across the back. Black, White or Grey. S, M or L.

#201 Or with the PC Star Logo Embroidery $35

C. **#400** Bike Shorts with Logo Patch Embroidery to match #200/201 above in Blk., Wht. or Grey. S, M or L $35

D. **#250** Leotard with embroidered PC Logo Patch in Blk., Wht. or Grey. S, M or L.

#251 Or with the PC Star Logo embroidery $35

E. **#450** Ankle pant with Logo Patch embroidery in Blk.,Wht. or Grey. S, M or L $35

F. **#300** Ladies Fitted Mini Tank with embroidered PC Logo Patch in Black or White. S, M or L.

#301 Or with the PC Star Logo embroidery $35

G. **#401** Drawstring Boxer Shorts with Logo Patch embroidery in Blk., Wht. or Grey. S, M or L..$30

H. **#305** Turtleneck Racerback Top with the PC Logo Patch embroidered on the back. In Blk. or Wht. S, M or L $45

I. **#302** All-Cotton Classic Tee-shirt with the PC Star Logo embroidery in Blk., Wht. or Grey S, M or L. $30

J. **#500** Outdoor Fleece Vest with PC Star Logo in Blk. or Grey.........................$70

ORDERING INFORMATION   mail orders to: **Physical Culture Activewear, Inc.** P.O. Box 3938 New York, NY 10185-3938
By Phone: For fast service call us at 1 212-245-5878. Have your Visa, Discover, or MasterCard and a completed order form ready for easy reference.
By Fax: Fax your completed order form to 1 212-581-1694 along with your credit card information and daytime phone number.
By Mail: Mail us a completed order form with your personal check, money order or credit card information.

---

24 HOUR SERVICE
Charge to my: ❑ VISA   ❑ MASTERCARD   ❑ DISCOVER
Acct #: _____ Exp: _____
Signature: _____
Charge by Phone Call: 1-212-245-5878 or Fax: 1-212-581-1694

Name: _____ Phone: _____
Address: _____
City: _____ State/Country: _____ Zip: _____
Please allow 2-4 weeks for delivery.   Photocopies of this form are acceptable.

ITEM NUMBER	DESCRIPTION	SIZE	COLOR	QTY. x PRICE =	AMOUNT
				SUBTOTAL	
				NY residents add 8.25% Sales Tax	
SHIPPING & HANDLING: For order totals up to $20.00 include $2.50; for totals $20.01 to $35.00 include $4.00; for totals $35.01 to $50.00 include $5.00 and for totals $50.01 & up include $6.00. FOREIGN ORDERS ADD AN ADDITIONAL $6.00.					
			Send check or money order in U.S. dollars for the TOTAL AMOUNT